The ZEN of Bowel Movements

A Spiritual Approach to Constipation

Kathy A. Price

Published by:

Rock Rose Publishing
P.O. Box 192
Santa Barbara, CA 93102

Rock Rose Publishing
P.O. Box 192
Santa Barbara, CA 93102

Printed in the United States of America

ISBN 0-9642906-6-9

Library of Congress Catalog Card Number:
95-70059

To Peter, Julie, Molly

and the Goddess

Table of Contents

I

Letting This Book Encourage You

Often the wisdom of the body clarifies the despair of the spirit.

- *Marion Woodman*

If you wish to know how you really stand spiritually, look about you at your environment, beginning with the body.

- *Emmet Fox*

It does not matter how slow you go as long as you do not stop.

- *Confucius*

We are living in a very exciting and powerful time . . . . We are, in fact, in the process of destroying our old world and building a new world in its place.

- *Shakti Gawain*

First off, "The Zen of Bowel Movements" is not a joke book. So if you were looking for even more jokes about bowel movements ("I won't offer you a stool when you come to visit," a furniture-maker friend said recently when I mentioned my book. Ha. Ha.), then you have your hands on the wrong book. Sorry. Put it back.

However, if you are constipated and tired of so-called remedies that never seem to cure your horrible problem, then you are holding the right book.

Actually, it's that very tendency to make jokes about bowel movements that makes this particular book so needed. Any of us who suffers from constipation—from the toxins cursing through our bodies as a result—doesn't need another joke. Oh sure, it's good to laugh. Happiness is certainly part of the solution. But jokes at our expense? Not here. Not now.

This book is based on a premise: We are constipated because our bodies are dutifully mirroring for us the dis-ease of our spirits. That disease I call holding back. As in holding back our true personalities, our talents, our vulnerable sides, our sacred feelings, our non-conformist thoughts, even our conformist thoughts.

Are you outwardly mild mannered, approval-seeking and even spiritually savvy? But inside do you hear the roar of a wild woman or man? The peep of a total geek? The silence of a bona fide recluse? Hey, it's just you and me here. Just tell the truth. Listen deeply. What do you hear? What is that stirring? If you have hidden the truth even from yourself, this book will help ferret it out.

Next question: Why are you going to work damned hard to find and release your true self? Because you are constipated! And you are miserable. And you don't want to be. The truth is, you are desperate. That's why you picked up this book. Good work already.

What else are we holding back? We are holding back our visions of the future, of what life could be like. We are holding back our terrifying opinions of the status quo.

We hold back our love, our tenderness, our softness. And why are we gripping these so tightly to our bosoms? Because it is dangerous to be authentic. It is not wanted in our society. Like your mother taught you, it's a good way to get your feelings hurt.

But you, dear desperate one, are going to come out of your false self, the one steeped in depression and negativity and anxiety, no matter what. And do you know why? Because you are constipated and you will do anything to get well. Underneath all the misery there is a wild river raging in your spirit that says "NO! This is not right for me! This sickness I will not have!"

I bet you've tried more remedies than you're willing to admit in mixed company. I know I have. Good. This book will work best for those who have tried all the laxatives, the dieter's tea, the colonics, the herbs, the yoga poses, and everything anyone else can think to sell us. If all these "cures" have failed you, then you are ready to rock and roll with this book.

You are ready because you know, deep down, the truth of your situation: If you heal your spirit, your body will reflect that health. Keep your soul clamped down and, well, you know what your body does.

You are going to come out of your misery. You have already started. You are going to release your authentic self. You are going to help save the world! And you won't be constipated anymore. Your bowel movements will be natural. And full. And beautiful. Every day.

How this Book is Arranged

This volume is meant to be used as a meditation book, to be read and contemplated a little bit at a time. However, you may want to start the book at the beginning and read right through to the end. Or, you might want to start at the end and read through to the beginning. Or, you may wish to open it at random spots and contemplate the messages there. Or, you may wish to search the table of contents for a chapter that calls to you.

What I am suggesting here is essentially the entire message of the book: You must find what works best for your unique self and do that. If the ideas you find here ring true inside, you are encouraged to go deeper into those concepts. But if these ideas sound like a bunch of bull, or sound dangerous, please get this book the heck out of your life as soon as possible.

As with most things, you may adore some of this book and abhor some of it. In that case, take what you like and leave the rest.

You may have bought the book because of the "Zen" in the title. You may wonder what the possible connection could be between your constipation and an ancient Eastern tradition. In a nutshell, Zen represents the awareness of spirit in everyday life. To see life as it really is. To see ourselves as we really are. This may be the beginning of a long and sometimes painful process of letting go of the lies and masks that once protected our true selves—but that now cause us deep dis-ease.

While this book is based on Zen principles, it does not contain specific directions on Zen meditation. If you wish to do that in a formal way, you will have to go elsewhere to get the instruction you desire. And you will not necessarily see the word "Zen" repeated in this book over and over again. But one does not need to say the word to live the practice.

The body of the work is organized in six sections, with three appendixes in the back. If you are especially curious about the physical manifestations of constipation, you may wish to turn straight to "Appendix A: An Odyssey Through Constipation Hell" and "Appendix B:

A Way of Letting Bowels Move." Together, these two chapters are the tale of my lifelong constipation, and of a smashed spirit, and of my transformation.

But here is a necessary warning: This book contains a suggested path only. The most important thing for you to do is take responsibility for finding your own way. The author is not responsible for your health or lack of it. Please don't do anything mentioned in this book without consulting your health professional. (Actually, consulting outside medical sources for this problem is exactly what we need to get away from. The answers are within. But I must suggest you consult your health professional to protect myself. Just use your best judgment and don't get hurt.)

In some ways of thinking, I am taking a big risk putting these suppositions out into the universe without an official license. But who gives a license in spiritual bowel management? It does not exist, and so I must claim myself an expert on my body. And you must claim yourself an expert on yours. For all my study on the subject—out of pure desperation, you can be sure—I have done enough work to have earned at least two doctorates.

May you have much success in finding your way to natural, fantastic bowel movements. Surely it is one of the great joys of life our creator intended for us. If you find this book useful, or if you have ideas of your own that are not covered here, please write. While this is a very private and individual situation, we are not alone. Many of us are engaged in the same search for bowel health.

As you will discover by reading this book, the search for natural bowel releases can be the cornerstone of an entire spiritual program.

Kathy A. Price
Santa Barbara, California

II

Letting the Earth Hold Us

This, then, is salvation: When we marvel at the beauty of created things and praise their beautiful Creator.

—Meister Eckhart

Zen is not some kind of excitement, but concentration on our usual everyday routine.

—Shunryu Suzuki

Chapter 1

Letting Our Bodies Teach Us

The soul loves the body.

—*Meister Eckhart*

At every moment, our bodies are continually responding to the messages from our minds. So what message is your mind giving your body?

—*Margo Adair*

The way to a beautiful, strong, healthy body is to start trusting yourself right now. . . . The body knows perfectly well what's good for it.

—*Shakti Gawain*

God does not despise what (God) has made, nor does (God) disdain to serve us in the simplest natural functions of our body.

—*Julian of Norwich*

Earth and heaven are in us.

—***Mahatma Ghandi***

Black folks find white folks afraid of their bodies. Blacks bring their bodies even to worship—especially to worship with.

—***Nathan Jones***

Do not disdain your body. For the soul is just as safe in its body as in the Kingdom of Heaven.

—***Mechtild of Magdeburg***

Our bodies are the manifestation of our consciousness in physical form.

—***Shakti Gawain***

Spiritual and religious traditions, when shaped by the feminine principle, affirm the cyclical phases of our lives and the wisdom each phase brings, the sacredness of our bodies and the body of the earth.

—***Patrice Wynne***

You are a principal work, a fragment of God. . . , you have in yourself a part of (God). Why then are you ignorant of your high birth?

—***Epicetus***

Every creature is a word of God and is a book about God.

—***Meister Eckhart***

To talk about God in relation to our sexuality means to be aware of love moving in us, for "in God we live and move and have our being."

—***Dorothee Soelle***

If life and the soul are sacred, the human body is sacred.
—*Walt Whitman*

To be humble means to be in touch with the earth, in touch with one's own earthiness, and to celebrate the blessing that our earthiness, our sensuality, and our passions are. To deny our earthiness is to bottle up deep and divine energies of creativity and imagination.
—*Matthew Fox*

Oh, to unleash my deep and raging passions! Yes! I want it! What does it take? I will work for it. Do these statements reveal your own true desires? To let your passionate self out of its prison? As it happens, we can look to our bodies for clues about our spirits.

If we think about it, what statement could hold more wisdom that "the mind/body connection?" How in the world could the mind and body not be connected? It's like talking about the root/trunk connection of a tree, or the leaf/branch connection. One does not thrive or wither without the other.

And yet much of the Western world speaks of this mind/body connection as if were a new-fangled idea, a New-Age thought.

But here's the truth, the way it's always been: The condition of our bodies are a testament to the condition of our minds, to the condition of our spirits. And perhaps that's why the wisdom of our sickened bodies is so difficult to accept and learn from—it exposes the deep sickness that we had felt could never be healed, the deep misery we hoped to keep as our own private secret. Maybe if we put on a good outer show the world won't know that we almost hate our very cells, that we don't feel welcome on this Earth, that we truly believe with every fiber of our beings that we are aberrations, mistakes.

Even now, with our desperation and our resolve to come out of our misery, and this book in our hands, we may want to deny this lifelong sickness of the spirit. It seems so impossible to change. Maybe I'll hold onto my mask of "I'm fine. How are You?" a little longer.

But guess what? The bad news is, if our bodies' conditions are any indication, the charade doesn't work. And that's the good news, really.

With our constipation—and our asthma, cancer, arthritis, acne, obesity, anorexia, infections, brittle fingernails, dull hair and/or a litany of other ailments—we are shown that we have great spiritual distress.

This is hard to admit, hard to embrace. But what is the alternative? We can spend our time, our money, our energy—our very lives—trying with futility to fix the outer symptoms. Or we can turn to our bodily dysfunctions as welcome, crystalline indicators of deeper issues and start right this moment to take the steps out of our misery.

We get much support in the former choice. Look at

the rich plastic surgeons, diet gurus, laxative companies, advertising agencies and television stations. Many, if not all, support big executive bank accounts and lavish lifestyles. Indeed, whole greed-driven industries depend on you and me being sick and spending our wages on "cures" that do not work. In this system, the salve sellers are guaranteed repeat customers, which everyone knows is key to more sales and more wealth.

All that being so, you and I don't have to participate. In this case, there are no victims, only volunteers. Through our own ignorance and laziness, we have rendered ourselves vulnerable, losers in this game we cannot win. We can't wait around for a referee to take us out of the ring, seeing that we are bloodied and bent. Pulling out of the madness is our job. It is our responsibility to say "Enough! I've had more than enough of this lie, this travesty to my body. And my deep wisdom. And my sense of self! I'm outta here!"

We can do it. We must. And once we do make that decision and begin to turn our faces away from those who do not have our best interests in mind, we begin to turn toward the light, toward the wisdom of our bodies, which have been patiently reflecting our spiritual maladies all along.

Once we start listening to our bodies, our healing has begun. Each malady has a message. We might not be able to heal from the malady right away, or even in this lifetime, but we can be aware of the wisdom of the truth.

We can love the messenger.

Why are our bodies overweight? Perhaps we are scared inside and are trying to create a layer of protection. Why are our bodies underweight? Perhaps we feel insignificant and worthless and want to take up less space. Why are we suffering from arthritis? Perhaps we harbor deep anger that seems impossible to release. Why do we have constipation? Perhaps we have a hard time letting go, a hard time being relaxed, a hard time trusting.

Now be careful here. The tendency is to blame ourselves for our physical maladies and feel that it's all our fault. That is not the message. Our physical maladies are not value judgments. They are thoughtful indicators of where we need to grow, of our learning curve. Of our edge, as they say in yoga class. We didn't choose to be sick in these ways. And even if we did—consciously or unconsciously—the time is now to read those symptoms like an instruction manual and begin to take deep action.

Our symptoms are like a guard standing alert on a hill to warn a peaceful tribal village of coming danger. Imagine that the guard starts waving a red flag to indicate danger is approaching. What should the tribe do? Would it be helpful to take the flag away? Incapacitate the guard? Slice away the hill where the guard stands? None of those actions would take care of the real problem—the approaching danger. That's what our physical maladies are for. They are like servant guards telling us that something is off kilter, something is amiss. Our constipation is a very clear indication that we are not letting life flow through us, that we are resisting. To surgically or chemically alter our bodies does not begin to heal the real cause of distress.

Surely our higher power did not bring us here so we could resist life. Surely our constipation is a clue to our deeper unhappiness. The constipation will begin to heal when the inner spiritual state begins to heal. We can begin today to find ways of letting go, to get the help we need to learn a new way of living. Our bodies will not let us rest until we do this. Our wise bodies will continue to reflect our spiritual state. This is the law of nature. There is no other way.

Write On:

Make a list of all your physical challenges, leaving space after each one. Then, letting your imagination go wild, list possible psychic and spiritual messages that your body could be sending you.

For example, my list would include toenail fungus, tendency toward overweight, constipation and keloids (scar tissue) on my shoulders. Under toenail fungus, I might guess that the message from my body could be: 1) a need to keep my foundation (moral and emotional) free from contaminants, or 2) to be careful with whom I mingle my energy (I caught this from an ex-boyfriend), or 3) I have a tendency to hide my defects, like toenail fungus under my socks and shoes.

Your musings on the message behind your physical challenges are there to serve you, to let you know where you might have the inclination to move in a certain way that maybe you don't need to go anymore.

Affirmation of Truth:

My body does not lie; it leads me to the truth.

Chapter 2

The Outrageous Ordinary

The religious is found in the everyday, the sacred in the profane.

—Heinrich Dumoulin

When something does not insist on being noticed, when we aren't grabbed by the collar or struck on the skull by a presence or an event, we take for granted the very things that most deserve our gratitude.

—Cynthia Ozick

It is extraordinary how extraordinary the ordinary person is.

—George F. Will

Any experience of reality is indescribable!

—R.D. Laing

Humankind cannot bear very much reality.

—*T.S. Eliot*

Never get so fascinated by the extraordinary that you forget the ordinary.

—*Magdalen Nabb*

In Buddhism there is no place for using effort. Just be ordinary and nothing special. Eat your food, move your bowels, pass water, and when you're tired go and lie down. The ignorant will laugh at me, but the wise will understand.

—*Rinzai*

I go about looking at horses and cattle. They eat grass, make love, work when they have to, bear their young. I am sick with envy of them.

—*Sherwood Anderson*

Monotony is the law of nature. Look at the monotonous manner in which the sun rises. The monotony of necessary occupations is exhilarating and life-giving.

—*Mahatma Ghandi*

I searched through rebellion, drugs, diets, mysticism, religions, intellectualism, and much more, only to begin to find . . . that truth is basically simple—and feels good, clean and right.

—*Chick Corea*

The aspects of things that are most important for us are hidden because of their simplicity and familiarity.

—*Wittgenstein*

God is in the details.

—*Mies Van Der Rohe*

Details are all there is.

—Maezumi

Most human beings have an almost infinite capacity for taking things for granted.

—Aldous Huxley

It is the familiar that usually eludes us in life. What is before our nose is what we see last.

—William Barrett

I prefer to explore the most intimate moments, the smaller, crystallized details we all hinge our lives on.

—Rita Dove

The fullness of joy is to behold God in everything.

—Julian of Norwich

How easy is it to get sucked into searching for the spectacular, the extraordinary, the stupendous. The modern world blasts us with a barrage of stimulus. The average Western citizen is daily exposed to thousands of images on television alone.

The communications revolution has cursed as well as blessed us. In our confusion, we may think we are missing something really meaningful right around the corner, on the next channel, something we must have before we can be happy.

What this chapter suggests is that a beautiful, miraculous life is already ours. All we need to do is see it, to slow down and contemplate the magnificence of a dew-laden leaf, the joy in a child's mind, the compassion in a dog's eyes, the peace in a oak tree. All these are our wealth, our abundance, our welcome-home gifts just for being born.

Perhaps this is easy for me to feel, writing this book at a bucolic Santa Barbara retreat center on a soft and silent September afternoon. On the other hand, no one forced me to be here. It was entirely my idea. My need.

We must acknowledge our need for simplicity, if that's what we need, and make arrangements to get it, to be away from phones and faxes and televisions and cars. And this doesn't have to cost us money. With a bit of creativity and a lot of persistence, there are ways to get the quiet we need and still have money for rent.

These days, it takes effort to slow our lives down. This wasn't such a challenge back when we lived on isolated farms and our main diversion was reading the Sears catalogue.

But s-l-o-w d-o-w-n is what we must do—filter out the excesses of the world in order to focus on what is meaningful. That's not to say we need to leave the world as we know it. But we must be in the world on our terms, getting what we need to be happy and whole in order to make our contribution.

This reverence of things ordinary includes appreciation for regular bowel movements. Many who have them take them for granted. They have other challenges in this lifetime. But for those of us who have struggled with constipation for years or decades, a robust bowel movement can be a most spectacular event. It's like a person who was born blind and got eye transplants at age 40. You can be sure she doesn't take the ability to see for granted the way I do.

And even if no one else in our social circle knows, or is too polite to admit, how full, natural bowel movements can fill us with unspeakable joy and peace, we who share this book can feel a deep kinship with each other. I am speaking your language, and you mine. I don't buy into a certain newspaper article about laxatives that said if one has too much of a fascination with bowel movements, one should see a psychologist. Well, I am extremely interested in bowel functions—mine in particular, yours by extension—and I consider myself extremely healthy. What do you think?

Consider this: An intimate, incredibly important function of our bodies has been—or is being—restored, healed, brought back to perfection. I say *hallelujah* sisters and brothers! Letting go of wastes may seem ordinary to some. But for us it is a major miracle on this Earth.

And Amen to that!

Write On:

Make a list of all the ordinary things in your life that are quite perfect. This could include your thick hair, the clean air in your town, the pretty blue tile in the bathroom, your talent for catching busses right on time, your capacity for listening to others.

Keep this list nearby and refer to it often. When you feel down, make a new list of ordinary miracles.

Affirmation of Truth:

Much is sheer perfection in my life, if I would only acknowledge it. I pause to notice my incredible bounty of gifts from the universe.

Chapter 3

Living a Simple, Sacred Life

We should make every effort to avoid the pressures and anxieties that fill most modern lives. The only way out is to consume less. Once we are able to live simply and happily, we are better able to help others.

—*Thich Nhat Hanh*

People love chopping wood. In this activity one immediately sees results.

—*Albert Einstein*

The more you have and the more you get, the more you have to look after. The more you might lose. Is that owning or being owned? But if you give up things, you can give up spending your life looking after things.

—*John Heider*

Beauty is all around us, but how many are blind to it! People take little pleasure in the natural and quiet and simple things of life.

—*Pablo Casals*

I have a simple philosophy: Fill what's empty. Empty what's full. Scratch where it itches.

—*Alice Roosevelt Longworth*

Every gesture is important. How we eat, how we put on our clothes, how we wash ourselves, how we go to the toilet, how we put our things away, how we act with other people, family, (spouse), work—how we are: totally, in every single gesture.

—*Taisen Deshimaru*

The ability to simplify means to eliminate the unnecessary so that the necessary may speak.

—*Hans Hoffman*

Possessions, outward success, publicity, luxury—to me these have always been contemptible. I believe that a simple and unassuming manner of life is best for everyone, best both for the body and the mind.

—*Albert Einstein*

One cannot collect all the beautiful shells on the beach, one can only collect a few.

—*Anne Morrow Lindbergh*

Put your heart, mind, intellect and soul even to your smallest acts. This is the secret of success.

—*Swami Sivananda*

There is more to life than increasing its speed.

—*Mahatma Ghandi*

Everybody seems to be in such a terrible rush today, anxious for greater developments and greater riches—so that our children have very little time with their parents. Parents have little time for each other, and in the home begins the disruption of the peace of the world.

—Mother Teresa

While washing the dishes one should only be washing the dishes, which means that while washing the dishes one should be completely aware of the fact that one is washing the dishes. At first glance, that might seem a little silly: why put so much stress on a simple thing? But that's precisely the point. The fact that I am standing there and washing these bowls is a wondrous reality. I'm being completely myself, following my breath, conscious of my presence, and conscious of my thoughts and actions. There's no way I can be tossed around mindlessly like a bottle slapped here and there on the waves.

—Thich Nhat Hanh

Is it so small a thing
To have enjoyed the sun
To have lived light in the spring
To have loved, to have thought, to have done?

—Matthew Arnold

We are lucky, in a way, to be living in this fast-paced world of more, more and more—more money, more meetings, more activities, more commitments, more status. We have taken this attitude to its limit and have discovered one thing: More is not the answer. Not when happiness, contentment and love are the quests.

And more confusion is certainly not the answer when a smoothly functioning body (which includes regular, natural and full bowel movements) is desperately sought. The body, which doesn't lie, is a great asset to us in determining how our lives need to change. When we are overly busy and our lives are overly complicated, our bodies get tied up in fear and our bowels won't move. We can stay busy and disregard this holy message. We can take laxatives for the rest of our unnatural lives.

Or, we can listen to this message and let it guide us.

The world we have known lately does not encourage us to have simple lives. In order for extremely money-rich people to get even more so, we must be turned into needy, discontented, consuming maniacs. If we feel the need for 100 pairs of shoes and 50 pairs of slacks, so much the better for profits. And bless those people for doing what they feel they must, what may be their truly spiritual path this lifetime. This is their right. But our responsibility is to find a way of being that is not harmful to ourselves or others or the Earth.

Actually, this trend toward a simpler life is already well into motion. But most of the attention is focused, in fear, on the disintegration of the old ways. As contemporary spiritual teacher Shakti Gawain says: "For many people, this time may be distressing, because the world situation and/or our personal lives may seem to be going from bad to worse. . . . The simple truth is that the old way of life that we have been following for centuries does not work."

Many forward-thinking companies are downsizing. Patagonia, a wildly successful Southern California clothing company, recently reduced its catalogue so that it now offers only two kinds of ski pants instead of five. As Patagonia founder and environmental activist Yvon Chouinard said, "Two types of ski pants to choose from are enough." Indeed. Looking ahead, he sees people losing their interest in spending money for the entertainment value of it.

These are wise thoughts for us all. For the truth is, simple living is so full of joy and beauty when we notice it that we can hardly stand the brightness. But it is all there, and mostly without cost: the sunrises and sunsets, the crashing waves, the caressing wind, the graceful movements of our minds, our surprising capacities for deep love, our very breath.

We can stop looking far away for the happiness we know, deep down, should be a part of our lives. That happiness is not "out there." It is inside us, in our appreciation for ourselves and for this world in which we live. The secret of the sacred is in the simple.

Write On:

Write out a list of your simple pleasures. Include

those you engage in daily, those in your past, and those you imagine are in your future. Perhaps a windy morning or evening fills you with some unspeakable awe. I remember a late morning in my childhood, lying on a green lawn, under the slight shade of a newly planted tree. The feeling I had of peace and safety stays with me decades later.

Make your own list as extensive as possible, and add to it later as memories and realizations come back. Keep your focus on this topic during a whole week, so you don't overlook those pleasures which are so easy to overlook, and yet so critical to happiness.

Affirmation of Truth

My simple life is a sacred life

Chapter 4

Rejoicing in the Physical World

Every grain of dust has a wonderful soul.

—*Joan Miro*

The day of my spiritual awakening was the day I saw—and I knew I saw—all things in God and God in all things.

—*Mechtild of Magdeburg*

Look. This is your world! You can't not look. There is no other world. This is your world; it is your feast. You inherited this; you inherited these eyeballs; you inherited this world of color. Look at the greatness of the whole thing. Look! Don't hesitate—look! Open your eyes. Don't blink, and look, look—look further.

—*Chogyam Trungpa*

Earth's crammed with heaven.

—Elizabeth Barrett Browning

It were happy if we studied nature more in natural things, and acted according to nature, whose rules are few, plain and reasonable.

—William Penn

Nature has no goal though she hath law.

—John Donne

The truth of a thing is the feel of it, not the think of it.

—Stanley Kubrick

The world is charged with the grandeur of God.

—Gerard Manly Hopkins

I believe in God, only I spell it nature.

—Frank Lloyd Wright

Wind moving through the grass so that the grass quivers. This moves me with an emotion I don't even understand.

—Katherine Mansfield

Holy persons draw to themselves all that is earthly.

—Hildegard of Bingen

Our faith imposes on us a right and duty to throw ourselves into the things of the earth.

—Teilhard de Chardin

The solution to my life occurred to me one evening while I was ironing a shirt.

—Alice Munro

Think with the whole body.

—Taisen Deshimaru

We know too much and feel too little.

—Bertrand Russell

I got the blues thinking of the future, so I left off and made some marmalade. It's amazing how it cheers one up to shred oranges and scrub the floor.

—D.H. Lawrence

We belong to the ground
It is our power
And we must stay close to it
or maybe we will get lost.

—Narritjin Maymuru Yirrkala
An Australian Aborigine

Everything that is in the heavens, on the earth, and under the earth, is penetrated with connectedness, penetrated with relatedness.

—Hildegard of Bingen

I been so busy thinking about (God) I never truly notice nothing God make. Not a blade of corn (how it do that?), not the color purple (where it come from?). Not the little wildflowers. Nothing.

—Alice Walker
"The Color Purple"

The natural world is a spiritual house. . . . (Humankind) walks there through forests of physical things that are also spiritual things, that watch (one) with affectionate looks.

—Charles Baudelaire

In music, in the sea, in a flower, in a leaf, in an act of kindness. . . , I see what people call God in all those things.

—***Pablo Casals***

Holy Mother Earth, the trees and all of Nature are witnesses of your thoughts and deeds.

—***Winnebago saying***
(American Indian)

Can we accept the great gift of our high births? For we have inherited a wonderful world. And we are meant to be here, in these physical bodies, on this physical Earth. This is not something to transcend. This is something to embrace.

We might also feel sad, seeing what the past 5,000 years of a dominator (rather than a cooperative) culture has done to the Earth, raping it of what once seemed like unlimited resources. Many today believe this way is coming to an end. As Monica Sjoo said in her book, "The Great Cosmic Mother," about this way of life, which is disrespectful of the Earth: "We must end it or it will end us."

Surely one way to end the rape of the Earth (and of its people) is to see and appreciate the full glory of the natural world. In general, patriarchal religions believe that only humans (sometimes only men!) have spirits and were born to dominate the Earth and all the animals and plants. Earlier pagan religions believed the Earth was itself a spiritual being and was to be worshiped.

During religious wars, millions of Earth-loving people, mostly women who were called witches, were burned, tortured and slaughtered. Some refer to the time as the Female Holocaust.

This horrific past is part of our mass consciousness. We're unconsciously terrified to love nature and the Earth. We are so frightened of just the word "witchcraft" that we don't know what it represents. We think it is the epitome of evil. But the truth is that witches were, and are, deeply connected with the Earth and its energies.

Nature is a great teacher for our lives. I sat by a river the other day and noticed how every tree and bush reaches for its true glory, taking into consideration all the factors of its environments—availability of sunlight, water and soil nutrients, and with respect for the season. Each tree strives to be its best, however scraggly, crooked or bent that might be. A tree doesn't refuse to try because conditions are challenging. A tree isn't poisoned with resentment because the bush across the river gets more sun. A tree doesn't spend half its energy judging the amount of water the river carries. A tree does its best, no matter what.

Of course, this Earth worship is not useful in religions were God is up in the sky somewhere and one has to go through religious men to get to "him." To these religions, the Earth is practically the enemy, the opposite of God, and certainly in the opposite direction. It's easy to see why we might be disconnected from the Earth, and then from our own natural bodies.

And, it's also easy to see why this system is coming to an end. As Episcopal priest and theologian Matthew Fox (who was kicked out of the Catholic Church) says in his books on creation spirituality, the Earth-based theologies are our future.

Of course, those of us who have despised our own bodies can understand the mass hatred of the Earth. Those of us who have been constipated and in pain can feel for the pain of our beautiful and scarred Earth.

The sickness of the body has its foundation on one basic lie: that there is something inherently wrong with us, that we are evil and flawed to the core. I felt that way for years, that I had serious DNA problems. Of course, this is tantamount to saying there is no loving spirit of the universe, no creator, that all is chaos without reason or love. But just one glance at this place should convince any awake person that something awesome and beyond out ability to comprehend runs this show.

As we become more aware of our spiritual natures, we will see that our bodies and the Earth that nurtures us are all holy beings. We are all manifestations of a creator which is generous and loving beyond belief.

When our bodies will not function, when our bowels will not move, that is a powerful message that we are not hearing the truth, that we are blocking out the love we were brought here to receive and to give. And it is our responsibility to hear this message and search for a solution.

Luckily, the answer most of the time is simply (but not always easily) to reject the lies and let the glory of our beings thrive in their intended, natural states of health. Healthy bowel movements are our divine right.

Write On:

List the physical things in the world that are wonderful beyond belief. Perhaps you are enthralled with the sun through leaves. Or with Rolex watches. Or with green salads. Really think hard to remember those things that move you, that delight you.

Then, make a list of your own body parts and functions that are spectacular. If you look in a book on the human body, you will be amazed at how the lungs work, how exactly the cells absorb oxygen and take it through the bloodstream to the extremities of our beings. Even if we are suffering from constipation, our bodies are probably more healthy than sick. How about the hair that grows on your legs just days after you shave them? Now that's persistence!

Affirmation of Truth

Full, healthy bowel movements are my divine right, and I am grateful for these most beautiful of happenings.

III

Letting Go Means Letting Be

You do not owe an atom of loyalty to anyone or anything in the universe except your own spiritual integrity.

—*Emmet Fox*

Chapter 5

Being Authentic

What I do is me. For that I came.

—Gerard Manly Hopkins

Be Yourself. Who else is more qualified?

—Frank J. Giblin II

If you can just observe what you are and move with it, then you will find that it is possible to go infinitely far.

—Krishnamurti

I too am born and grown to be this thing only; to be Anna in the world.

—Anna Rydstedt-Dannstedt

I can't write a book commensurate with Shakespeare, but I can write a book by me.

—Sir Walter Raleigh

In the world to come they will not ask me, "Why were you not Moses?" They will ask me, "Why were you not Zusya?"

—Zusya of Hanipoli

Among the most remarkable features characterizing Zen we find these: spirituality, directness of expression, disregard of form or conventionalism, and frequently an almost wanton delight in going astray from respectability.

—D.T. Suzuki

I like being unconventional.

—Florence Griffith-Joyner

We must be true inside, true to ourselves, before we can know a truth that is outside us.

—Thomas Merton

The greatest danger, that of losing one's own self, may pass off quietly as if it were nothing; every other loss, that of an arm, a leg, five dollars, etc., is sure to be noticed.

—Soren Kierkegaard

The main thing in life is to not be afraid of being human.

—Pablo Casals

The moral deteriorations attendant on a false and shallow life are among the most pitiable wrongs that mortals suffer.

—Nathaniel Hawthorne

Being entirely honest with oneself is a good exercise.

—Sigmund Freud

Our entire life, with our fine moral code and our precious freedom, consists ultimately in accepting ourselves as we are.

—Jean Anouilh

You just have to be real—to yourself.

—Shakti Gawain

There is no ache more
Deadly than the striving to be oneself.

—Yevgenly Vinokurov

For have you not perceived that imitations, whether of bodily gestures, tones of voice, or modes of thought, if they be persevered in from an early age, are apt to grow into habits and a second nature?

—Plato

Take the place and attitude to which you see your unquestionable right, and all (people) acquiesce.

—Ralph Waldo Emerson

Change only occurs when one becomes what she is, not when she tries to become what she is not.

—Ruth P. Freedman

Cherish forever what makes you unique, 'cause you're really a yawn if it goes!

—Bette Midler

The question is laid out
For each of us to ask:
Whether to hold on
Or to drop the mask.

—Martha Boesing

Freedom means the right to be different, the right to be oneself.

—Ira Einstein

If there is any peace, it will come through being, not having.

—Henry Miller

Until you make peace with who you are, you'll never be content with what you have.

—Doris Mortman

The most exhausting thing in life is being insincere.

—Anne Morrow Lindbergh

There never were, since the creation of the world, two cases exactly parallel.

—Lord Chesterfield

If we all pulled in one direction, the world would keel over.

—Yiddish Proverb

What could prevent full, natural bowel movements more than the never-ceasing struggle to be that which we are not? The exhausting effort of trying to be some false self that our mind or society tells us we must be causes the guts and bowels to rebel, locking up like a put bull's jaws. "No!" our bodies say. "I won't condone this lunacy. I rebel!" I spent my early years worried that I would never be "normal." That I would never fit in. And my body was tightened up in fear of this.

Actually, this sickness of the body is our greatest blessing, a beacon of a serious and deep malady of the spirit. Our bodies are simply a physical manifestation of what's really going on. In our society, there are so many of us drowning in deep fear and massive resentment, who are not feeling free enough to really give of our true selves. Unfortunately, many of these people seem to be making television shows and commercials. And so their fears and discontentments spread like airwave-borne viruses to the rest of us.

This malcontentedness is so widespread in our culture that when we see truly happy, spontaneous, creative people, some try to destroy them, to silence them. This is because they reawaken in us our own powerful, never-ceasing desire to be free. This is part of the reason sick adults abuse beautiful, innocent children.

We must not let the sickness of the world destroy us. We must protect ourselves from life-draining people and environments and go inside ourselves for the truth. That is the purpose of meditation, to feel inside the quiet of ourselves what is the truth. The truth is that when the false, strained, plastic personality is removed, we are full of love and compassion, full of creativity and true joy. And when our spirits are aligned with the truth, our bodies just naturally begin to function properly, letting go of their wastes in a sweet and gentle way.

Of course, it takes a while to get comfortable with

being authentic, to having spontaneous actions that are not rehearsed and premeditated. In my own life of openness, I have been disrespected by those who would have me be more contained, more controlled. I have been looked down upon, and frowned upon, and talked about as crazy behind my back. So we not only must embrace our true selves, but we must resist those who would have us be dead inside.

For those of us who want to predict and control every situation, being authentic can bring unwanted, unplanned-for consequences. For in order to be authentic and move with our feelings, however wild and surprising, things do not always go as we think is best. However, the up side is that life becomes exciting. Everything changes and we change, too. We can have faith in the basic goodness of the universe, or be open to that possibility, and with searching and quiet reflection we can see how a thing was really for the best, after all.

It's a wild ride to be authentic. And the Earth is crying out for us to come out from behind our masks and be ourselves. Does this world need another fake personality? Another self-abandoning, discontent, greedy consumer? When we become more of who we truly are, we don't fall so easily into categories. We start to lose track of who we are, of who we are supposed to be. And this can be disconcerting—for us, for our families, friends and employers.

But what is driving us toward facing these changes

is a deep, serious desire to have a healthy body and full, natural bowel movements. If this desire is strong enough, we will not fail.

Write On:

Make a list of the ways you are truly unique. Include all the things you suspect might possibly be unique, those things you would be embarrassed to tell another person in case they weren't really unique or interesting.

My list would include my desire for a lot of alone time, my dislike of representational art, my love for contemporary art, my penchant for living in unusual homes (a caboose, for example).

Let this list evolve over a period of time, adding to it when people comment on something unique about you, or when you have a sudden realization that some part of you seems to be at odds with the rest of your culture. Don't judge what makes you unique. Just get it down on paper. Document it.

Affirmation of Truth

When people say I am "one in a million," I smile, and know that it is true.

Chapter 6

Keeping Outside Images in Their Place

You were once wild here. Don't let them tame you!

—Isadora Duncan

We would have much peace if we would not busy ourselves with the sayings and doings of others.

—Thomas A. Kempis

Let me listen to me and not to them.

—Gertrude Stein

Cursed be the social lies that warp us from the living truth.

—Alfred Lord Tennyson

One does not have to believe everything one hears.

—Cicero

What I must do is all that concerns me—not what people think.

—Ralph Waldo Emerson

You have the witness of Truth within yourself. You are no longer dependent upon the word of somebody else; you know for yourself; and this is the only authority worth having.

—Emmet Fox

What difference does it make how I am treated by life? My real life is within.

—Angela L. Wozniak

Everything intercepts us from ourselves.

—Ralph Waldo Emerson

We are all geniuses—each in our own unique way. We will discover the nature of our particular genius when we stop trying to conform to our own or other people's models.

—Shakti Gawain

I am more involved in unlearning than learning. I'm having to unlearn all the garbage that people have laid on me.

—Leo Buscaglia

Once in a while it really hits people that they don't have to experience the world in the way they have been told to.

—Alan Keightley

There is after all no obligation to answer to every passing fool according to (his or her) folly.

—Elias Canetti

Wonder of wonders! Intrinsically all living beings are Buddhas, endowed with wisdom and virtue, but because (people's) minds have become inverted through delusive thinking they fail to perceive this.

—Gautama the Buddha

If you follow the present-day world, you will turn your back on the Way; if you would not turn your back on the Way, do not follow the world.

—Takuan

There is no reality except the one contained within us. That is why so many people live such an unreal life. They take the images outside them for reality and never allow the world within to assert itself.

—Herman Hesse

I was raised to sense what someone wanted me to be and be that kind of person. It took me along time not to judge myself through someone else's eyes.

—Sally Field

Whatever course you decide upon, there is always someone to tell you you are wrong. There are always difficulties arising which tempt you to believe that your critics are right.

—Ralph Waldo Emerson

The dogs bark but the caravan moves on.

—Arabic Proverb

When she stopped conforming to the conventional picture of femininity she finally began to enjoy being a woman.

—*Betty Friedan*

Power is the strength and the ability to see yourself through your own eyes and not through the eyes of another.

—*Agnes Whistling Elk*

It's no wonder so many recovery programs for co-dependents have sprung up in the past decade; we have become so fused to each other that we don't know where one person leaves off and the next person begins.

If we tend toward co-dependency, it's easy to see how we got that way in the first place. As we have sliced away unacceptable parts of ourselves, ignored our deepest voices, we have become lonely and scared. And so we cling to others for our very lives, talking all the while about interdependence and sisterly/brotherly love. The truth is, we have been lost and we are looking for others to lead us home. But this is impossible, because the home we are looking for, as we peer far out into the distance, is inside of our own selves.

But outside images have conspired to make us lose touch with our centers, to blot out the truth of our beings. And when our guts are clenched in denial, we are constipated, unable to allow any form of truth to move through us.

One big offender is turning us away from ourselves, as has been mentioned before in this book, is advertising, especially television advertising. In order to sell their products, advertisers must encourage us to feel that we are defective and in need of an outside fix. It does not benefit advertisers—and their stooges, television producers—when we feel whole and complete and satisfied. For if we do, we cease to consume at a rate that keeps them hauling in the riches. As one wealthy company president said recently, "consumer confidence" is the key to revitalizing the economy. But it's consumer craving, consumer covetousness that he really wants. After all, truly confident consumers do not need vaginal deodorant, mouthwash, expensive liquors, beer parties and prestige automobiles.

Now I'm not advocating a massive, organized campaign to stamp out business and reasonable profits. Instead I am offering a simple suggestion—from myself in this moment on a crisp October morning, to you in the moment you are reading this passage: Be yourself, accept yourself, celebrate your truth. Like Mother Teresa says: "Do not wait for leaders. Do it all alone, person to person."

Many today are suggesting we stop submitting ourselves to the commercial propaganda that needs us to turn away from our own selves for its survival—not ours. Basically, it comes down to this: It's me or the ads. Do I serve them or do I serve myself and the world? Do

I survive and thrive, or do they? In the long run, if I don't survive, then all is for naught anyway.

In our culture, we must search diligently to find support for our mission of protecting ourselves from negative images. Every now and again, and more and more, we find a person who does not watch television, who doesn't even own a television. If Karl Marx were alive today, he would say that television has taken over from religion as the opiate of the masses. The pervasiveness of television is astounding. We are a nation of addicts in denial. And our children are the most tender victims.

But how will we know what is going on in the world without TV? First of all, what's going on in the world is not necessarily reflected on TV. The main purpose of TV is to entertain, to draw us away from our true selves. What we want is to be informed. That can be done with newspapers, where we can be selective about what we ingest. Newspapers don't realistically reflect what's going on in the world, either, but at least we are not hapless receivers of images. We are in control of when we turn the page or when we linger on a story.

As we recover more and more of ourselves, we become more deeply sensitive, more deeply aware. And so we must be even more careful about what we allow into our realm. For me, if I choose to expose myself to very powerful and carefully constructed commercials whose aim is to convince me of my neediness, my true self will wisely start to shut down, to go into hiding like it did when I was small child. And the constipation will return. Yuck!

Tragically, children have very little to say about their environments. The average child in the United States is subjected to more than 25 hours a week of TV images! Can you imagine how many murders and infidelities that includes? We are creating a generation of lost people who will surely have digestive problems as a result. This is good news for manufacturers of laxatives, but not good news for us.

The truth is, we are meant to be happy, to feel good and clean inside, and to have wonderful bowel movements. When outside images don't contribute to those natural states of well-being, we need to eliminate those images.

Few struggles will be as constant as keeping other people's opinions about us from affecting us, changing us, stifling us, destroying us. But the price we pay for not mustering the courage to become ourselves is constipation—spiritual, emotional and physical. The trouble is, the world can ill-afford to lose the real us. We were born here because we are needed here.

Write on:

Draw a large circle on a piece of paper. Make the circle thick, like a wall. Inside the circle put your name, and those people and influences that are good for you, that encourage you to become yourself even more deeply. This could include friends, spiritual counselors, your dog or cat, a kindly relative. It could also include movies by certain directors, publications that nurture and affirm you, practices like yoga that bring you closer home.

Outside of the circle, put those people and things that are bad for you. Certain people, for instance, criticize everything we do. Write down their names. Others drain our energy by talking about their own dramas all the time. Also, certain media is toxic for us. Maybe certain towns or states are draining for us. Write down everything and everyone who has a bad influence on you.

Post this drawing where you can see it. Add to it, amend it. It should be an evolving, fluid guide for you. And when one of those toxic, draining people or things comes near you, put up a psychological wall and keep their toxic gasses out.

Affirmation of Truth:

I preserve my good health—spiritually, physically, emotionally and mentally—by shielding myself from images that hurt my self-image. I protect myself and I thrive; it is my nature to thrive.

Chapter 7

Getting Support for Who We Are

One is taught by experience to put a premium on those few people who can appreciate you for what you are.

—*Gail Goodwin*

Friendships that work are relationships in which (people) help each other to belong to themselves.

—*Louise Bernikow*

As you continue to follow your path, you will increasingly attract people who like you as you are and want to relate to you in a new way.

—*Shakti Gawain*

The highest compact we can make with our fellow is, let there be truth between us two forevermore.

—*Ralph Waldo Emerson*

I will love you no matter what. I will love you if you are stupid, if you slip and fall on your face, if you do the wrong thing, if you make mistakes, if you behave like a human being—I will love you no matter.

—*Leo Buscaglia*

I get by with a little help from my friends.

—*John Lennon and Paul McCartney*

Avoid friends and followers who are detrimental to thy peace of mind and spiritual growth.

—*Tibetan Rosary of Precious Gems*

If I am too strong for some people, that's their problem.

—*Glenda Jackson*

Walk with the wise and be wise; mix with the stupid and be misled.

—*Proverbs*

That's the risk you take if you change; that the people you've been involved with won't like the new you. But other people who do will come along.

—*Lisa Alther*

Simply because we follow our own true selves doesn't mean we must be hermits. It's true that we want to rid our lives of those people and influences that conspire to destroy us. That is necessary. We must make room for those people who love us unconditionally to come into our lives.

Incidentally, this is not a judgment call on those people who drain our energies, who leave us feeling dirty, rejected and weak. I consider myself a tolerant, kind person, but there are people I simply can't stand to be around. I would encourage those people to stay away from me and not try to win me over. It's not worth it. I know, I've tried many times in the past to win people over.

Just show me a room with 300 people who adore me and one who despises me, and I would in the past go straight to that one. Why waste time with the others? They are already convinced. This one is my challenge. And anyway, those who don't support me also don't expect much of me. Those who love me expect me to be wonderful. And that's a burden. So we can see why we might be drawn to those we can't convince.

And I have found plenty of people who don't approve of me. Now, I stay as far away from those people as possible. Even Mother Teresa has her critics (she is totally co-dependent, some say. She's a jet-setter). Even Jesus wasn't exactly liked by all.

Think for a moment of your own early life and the people who have totally delighted in you. It seems that each of us are blessed with a certain number of fans—maybe a doting grandmother, a supportive teacher, a neighbor who thought you were just the most wonderful person, and seemingly for no reason at all.

That's what we're looking for here—people who totally love us for no rhyme nor reason, people who are on our side, no matter what, who believe we are magnificent without us having to perform any tricks or do gymnastics. We can have that. We must have that. But we need to make room for it, we need to open like a flower to the sun of kind people, to make room for that kind of experience. Moving toward love is a choice.

The fear, of course, is that once we kick the negative, energy-sapping people out of our lives, we will have no one. No wonderfully supportive people will materialize and we will be alone and lonely.

And so we stay hooked up with people who have a deep distaste for us. It's like the battered wife whose self-esteem is so low from the abuse that she feels unworthy of any other type of experience.

Often these scornful people remind us of family members who once tried to smash our spirits. We stay because it feels familiar. (Here's a tip: When making a new friend, if they have a habit of saying, "Shame on you," even in jest, best reconsider the friendship. Shame-based people have unlimited capacity to make us feel bad.)

But we are going to move beyond the surface familiarity of shame to what's truly familiar deep inside us—our truly authentic self being expressed and then cherished in this world. That is the great benefit of being human. We have the capacity to choose.

And this is what leads us to truly healthy, happy bodies and full, abundant bowel movements. We can remember that our natural state is health and love, and we can choose people who already see that in us. I know people who are so blinded by the good side of me that they don't see anything else about me, and if they do, they tell me lovingly. With support, we grow into our rightful glory. Again, we must be very careful who we allow into our presence. If someone sees the negative in everything, avoid them. Stick with people who honor this miracle we are all involved in. Your life—and your full bowel movements—depend on it.

Write On:

Make a list of people who have truly loved you and supported you. Write down, as completely as you can, the incidents when these people were there for you. Try to remember exactly your feelings and their actions.

I remember one time when I fell off a motorcycle and my genetic family stood on a hillside and laughed at me.

But my sister's boyfriend came running down the hill to hug me and ask me if I was OK. A memory of an angel like that is especially meaningful to heal the hurt of the incident as a whole.

Make your own list of angels and incidents as robust as possible. Afterward, take in the whole list and all your angels. Let the whole picture wash over you like you were being baptized in love.

Affirmation of Truth:

I have been loved and supported by certain people my whole life. I hold them up to the light and thank them. And I am loved by God, by the Goddess and by the Earth. I am exactly what they had in mind when they created people.

Chapter 8

Being Ourselves Is Walking With Courage

Better to die on your feet than live on your knees.
—Dolores Ibarruri

And the trouble is, if you don't risk anything, you risk even more.
—Erica Jong

Let us move on, and step out boldly, though it be into the night, and we can scarcely see the way.
—Charles B. Newcomb

Courage is the price that life exacts for granting peace.
—Amelia Earhart

There have been (people) in the past far more daring than we would need to be now, who ventured all and gained a little, but survived after all.

—Germaine Greer

I have accepted fear as a part of life—specifically the fear of change. I have gone ahead despite the pounding in the heart that says: turn back.

—Erica Jong

It's easy to be independent when you've got money. But to be independent when you haven't got a thing—that's the Lord's test.

—Mahalia Jackson

Everyone has talent. What is rare is to follow the talent to the dark place where it leads.

—Erica Jong

Woman must not accept; she must challenge. She must not be awed by that which has been built up around her; she must reverence that woman in her which struggles for expression.

—Margaret Sanger

Courage is fear that has said its prayers.

—Anonymous

Risk! Risk anything! Do the hardest thing on Earth for you. Act for yourself. Face the truth.

—Katherine Mansfield

Originality is unexplored territory. You get there by carrying a canoe—you can't take a taxi.

—Alan Alda

Who's not sat tense before (one's) own heart's curtain?

—Rainer Maria Rilke

Courage is resistance to fear, mastery of fear—not absence of fear.

—Mark Twain

Nobody told me how hard and lonely change is.

—Joan Gilbertson

How does it feel
To be on your own
With no direction home
Like a complete unknown
Like a rolling stone?

—Bob Dylan

i can't go on...
i really
can't go on
i swear
i can't go on
so
i guess
i'll get up
and go on

—Dory Previn

You must do the thing you think you cannot do.

—Eleanor Roosevelt

One doesn't discover new lands without consenting to lose sight of the shore for a very long time.

—Andre Gide

It is impossible, I think, taking our nature into consideration, that anyone who fails to realize that he or she is favored by God should have the courage necessary for doing great things.

—*St. Teresa of Avila*

People wish to learn to swim and at the same time to keep one foot on the ground.

—*Marcel Proust*

Better hazard once than always be in fear.

—*Thomas Fuller*

One happy benefit of claiming and championing our true selves can be a body that is humming and flowing along in concert with our spirits. And full bowel movements are part of that gift, as well as good self-esteem and a chance to contribute qualities that this world desperately needs.

Still, to search for our true selves is a very scary deal. What if I don't like my true self? What if you don't like me? I think maybe if I keep my real and vulnerable self, however inadequate it is, hidden behind a pleasing facade, then maybe I won't get hurt. Some of us found out as kids that to tell anyone of our deepest passions was to open ourselves up to be hurt later on. How many parents have discovered what the child really loves, only to take that away as punishment? At the time, it was better to keep the truth hidden, first from you, and then from myself. Soon, the memory of my authentic self becomes a dim, foggy memory.

To enter the search for our true selves is to navigate uncharted rivers—perhaps with critics on the shore, shouting out their displeasure with us, their fear for us, their terror of ever doing it themselves. Many of us will be tempted to give up the quest, put our boat into storage and plop ourselves in front of the TV for the rest of eternity.

Of course, this will not work for us. We will suffer the symptoms of living half a life. We will be constipated on all levels. However, if we would rather pay the price for what seems like safety—the heavy price of spiritual, emotional and physical illness—then we should put this book down and forget the whole thing. We all choose one way because we don't think we can survive the alternatives. Maybe now is not the right time for our search. Maybe later will be a better time. And maybe not. After all, we don't pick up a book like this because we want to stay in our misery.

If we do decide to go for it and expose our real selves to the light of day, we will do so with mighty souls beside us, with peers who can laugh with us and comfort us and challenge, love and respect us.

It's fun and helpful to watch other unique souls who have braved the journey within, and especially with those detractors shouting from the shore. I stand in awe of entertainer Bette Midler, writer Ray Bradbury, attorney Gloria Allred, singer Michael Jackson—all of them strange and wonderful and powerful, tremendous gifts to this planet.

It's tempting to think that we can only become our fully realized selves if everyone in the universe gives us a helping hand, lifting us up to our rightful place. But we don't need everyone. First, we need ourselves on our sides. Then, the help we need from a few supportive friends will naturally come our way. Our approval of ourselves will draw people to us who agree with us.

As we recover our truest selves from their hiding places, many are standing by, cheering us along, dizzy with excitement at the exotic dishes we will bring to the table. It's that excitement inside us—for our own journey and the journeys of others—that helps our bodies function and eliminate properly.

And whatever our ages or conditions, it's not too late to push off from the shore. As the English like to say: "It is better to begin in the evening than not at all."

Write On:

Make a list of the times you have acted with true courage that came from within yourself. This could be something you did for yourself, or for another person. And these acts don't need to be front-page news.

On my list is a time when I was at a meeting and an elderly woman came to the doorway. I could see that all the chairs were taken, and that if she was to sit down, somebody needed to get her a chair. Because I was so shy at the time, it was a really courageous act for me to get up, walk across the room, and get a chair for her. But I did it. I saw what needed to be done, and I was the one called to do it. This took courage for me to act.

Nowadays, these kinds of acts come more easily for me, and my courageous acts are of a different nature. But then, it was full-tilt courage.

Make your own list as full as possible. Read the whole list over several times. Add to it as memories come to you. We probably have been more courageous than we realize.

Affirmation of Truth:

I have been acting with courage in my whole life, and I continue to do so. I embrace my true self with the greatest courage of all.

IV

Letting Silence Speak

I think I must. . . be quiet so that my children can hear the Sound of Creation and dance the dance that is in them.

—*Russell Hoban*

Chapter 9

Taking Time for Quiet

All miseries derive from not being able to sit quietly in a room alone.

—*Blaise Pascal*

It is universally admitted that there is a natural healing power resident in the body. . . . Many people have learned to relax and to keep quiet like animals, giving nature a free opportunity to heal their maladies.

—*Horatio W. Dresser*

Nothing in all creation is so like God as stillness.

—*Meister Eckhart*

We need time to dream, time to remember, and time to reach the infinite. Time to be.

—*Gladys Taber*

Actually, these are among the most important times in one's life, when one is alone. Certain springs are tapped only when we are alone. The artist knows (s/he) must be alone to create; the writer, to work out (her/his) thoughts; the musician, to compose; the saint, to pray.

—*Anne Morrow Lindbergh*

God is the friend of silence. We need to find God, but we cannot find (God) in noise or excitement.

—*Mother Teresa*

Be still and listen to the stillness within.

—*Darlene Larson Jenks*

Endless drama. . . clouds consciousness. Too much noise overwhelms the senses. Continual input obscures genuine insight. Do not substitute sensationalism for learning. Allow regular time for silent reflection. Turn inward and digest what has happened.

—*Shakti Gawain*

To live a spiritual life, we must first find the courage to enter into the desert of loneliness and to change it by gentle and persistent efforts into a garden of solitude.

—*Henri J.M. Nouwen*

Be able to be alone. Lose not the advantage of solitude.

—*Sir Thomas Browne*

Solitude is bearable only with God.

—*Andre Gide*

I used to believe that anything was better than nothing. Now I know that sometimes nothing is better.

—*Glenda Jackson*

You do not need to leave your room. Remain sitting at your table and listen. Do not even listen, simply wait. Do not even wait, be quite still and solitary. The world will freely offer itself to you to be unmasked, it has no choice, it will roll in ecstasy at your feet.

—Franz Kafka

All the masters tell us that the reality of life—which our noisy waking consciousness prevents us from hearing—speaks to us chiefly in silence.

—Karlfried Graf Durckheim

Silence is the perfectest herald of joy; I were but little happy if I could say how much.

—William Shakespeare

Solitude is un-American.

—Erica Jong

What a lovely surprise to discover how un-lonely being alone can be.

—Ellen Burstyn

Fond as we are of our loved ones, there comes at times during their absence an unexplained peace.

—Anne Shaw

Haste, haste has no blessing.

—Swahili Proverb

Taking quiet time may seem like a luxury to many in this hectic world. But for those of us who suffer from chronic constipation, quiet time is necessary. The truth is, our bodies want to eliminate, to function in a way that keeps us cleaned out and detoxified. But habits of constant motion can work against that. We need exercise, to be sure, but we also need times of serenity.

Even in the most "enlightened" households, quiet time may be neglected in favor of other healing activities: listening to self-improvement or spiritual tapes, playing New Age music, sharing feelings with loved ones, chanting, singing, praying. And the list goes on. While all of these are valuable in their own ways, they may not allow us to really let go and observe the universe quietly moving within us. Part of what got us into this fix was trying to control everything. This is not the answer to this problem. A better remedy is letting ourselves be held and loved by the universe. As one man once told me when I was in early recovery, "You don't have to do anything. You're already magnificent."

Of course, this is where meditation comes in. If we are already meditators, congratulations to us. Hopefully we can do our meditation in the morning, which seems to be a time most human bodies want to eliminate. And hopefully, we can choose a meditation that has a foundation in what is natural, one that doesn't ask us to strain for something artificial (like breathing in a particular way or forcing our minds into certain patterns). Just remember that the goal here is to relax and let go, so we should find a meditation that supports that.

If we are not already meditators, we are in for a

wonderful experience. This could be what we've been looking for in all our therapies and self-improvement strategies. For many of us, meditation works best if we have willingly, willfully cleared out some of the garbage of the past through counseling and support groups. But after that work is done, there is another level to which we can travel. And that is to a deep acceptance of our true selves, of our bodies, of our very cells. Few things contribute to lovely bowel movements more than a deep love and approval for our physical being. And we don't get there by trying to change nature, by getting plastic surgery, by telling ourselves we are something we are not. We get there in meditation, in quiet time where we are perfectly OK in that moment.

There is good reason for making time for quiet in the morning. For those of us predisposed toward constipation, the stress and strain of our lives is reflected in our bodies (as are all our mental, emotional and spiritual states) by a tightening up of our internal organs. It's only natural, actually, that we should tense up when faced with modern life. This is a very complex and overwhelming world. But because we want more out of life than constipation, we must find ways out of our illness. When we can meditate early in the day, we practice getting in tune with the universe, which saves us time and energy later in the day when we aren't swimming against the truth, but are in the flow of the river of life.

All this may sound spacey and New Agey. But if

you suffer from constipation the way I have suffered from constipation, you stand willing to try anything to come out of your misery. Just do it. Try different meditation techniques, hook yourself up to a meditation teacher you feel good about, and learn to let go from the inside. You will be amazed at the results.

Write On:

Before writing, just sit quietly for a few minutes and notice the sensations in your body. Starting with your head, notice how your scalp feels. Do you detect an itch? Wind against your hair? A lightness? A heaviness? Just notice. Then, moving down your body, area by area, notice the sensations without judgment, without analysis. Just notice. How many sounds do you hear? Is one part of your body cooler or warmer than the others? Is there a scent in the air? Just notice.

Now write out your desire to spend time in mediation. Make it in the form of a prayer, if you wish. Write out the perfect scenario in which you could have the quiet time you need.

Affirmation of Truth:

In quite time with myself, I more clearly see the beauty and rightness of who I am. And, the answers I seek come to me in the quiet. Time spent with me is a priority.

Chapter 10

Taking Time to Know Our Inner Selves

Resolve to find thyself.

—***Matthew Arnold***

It all starts with self-reflection. Then you can know and emphasize more profoundly with someone else.

—***Shirley MacLaine***

Knowing others is wisdom. Knowing yourself is Enlightenment.

—***Lao Tzu***

I observe myself and so I come to know others.

—***Lao Tzu***

We carry our homes within us which enable us to fly.

—John Cage

To live is to be slowly born.

—Antoine de Saint-Exupery

When one is a stranger to oneself then one is estranged from others too.

—Anne Morrow Lindbergh

Inside myself is a place where I live alone, and that's where you renew your springs that never dry up.

—Pearl S. Buck

When we are unable to find tranquillity within ourselves, it is useless to seek it elsewhere.

—Francois de La Rochefoucauld

We are the hero of our own story.

—Mary McCarthy

Whatever I want to express in its truest meaning must emerge from within me and pass through an inner form. It cannot come from outside to the inside but must emerge from within.

—Meister Eckhart

We are stardust
We are golden
And we've got to get ourselves
Back to the garden.

—Joni Mitchell

Outside show is a poor substitute for inner worth.

—Aesop

I myself believe that the evidence for God lies primarily in inner personal experience.

—*William James*

My true relationship is my relationship with myself—all others are simply mirrors of it.

—*Shakti Gawain*

Everyone should feel as an artist does. Everyone should be free to let his or her inner mind speak to her. And everyone is an artist when she does this.

—*Kenji Miyazawa*

There is no need to run outside
For better seeing. . .
. . . Rather abide
At the center of your being;
For the more you leave it, the less you learn.
Search your heart and see. . .
The way to do is to be.

—*Lao Tzu*

If you do not express your own original ideas, if you do not listen to your own being, you will have betrayed yourself.

—*Rollo May*

Show me someone not full of herself and I'll show you a hungry person.

—*Nikki Giovanni*

The time is at hand when the voices of the feminine mystique can no longer drown out the inner voice that is driving women to become complete.

—*Betty Friedan*

How many times have you tried to shield yourself by reading the newspaper, watching television, or just spacing out? That is the $64,000 question: how much have you connected with yourself at all in your whole life?

—*Chogyam Trungpa*

"Living in the forest" would mean sinking into one's innermost nature and finding out what it feels like.

—*Marie-Louise von Frantz*

It's ironic, but until you can free those final monsters within the jungle of yourself, your life, your soul is up for grabs.

—*Rona Barrett*

This business of taking the time to know our inner selves can be terrifying. What if we're as boring as we fear? What if we're as inconsequential as the world makes us out to be? What if there's much less to us than we hoped? What if we're mad, demented, unacceptable, fatally flawed? These fears are widespread and pervasive. Especially if we live in a dream world of fantasy, fiction and escapism, we will be afraid to face what the truth may turn out to be.

But a fantasy world, especially one created by imaginations other than our own, does not serve those of us who are constipated. While our heads are in a made-up world, our true selves are being held captive inside.

Actually, it takes a lot of energy to hold our real selves back. And tight bowels are just a mirror of that holding back. Our wise bodies are showing us graphically the nature of our misery. To allow the true self to emerge is the key step on the path toward a fully functioning body, where letting go is easy.

The predicament of living false lives started for many of us in childhood, when we wisely suppressed those parts of us that were unacceptable to our caretakers, and adopted those ways of being which received approval. How could we have done differently? When we are totally dependent on someone for our survival, we do what is necessary to maintain that. Anything else would be suicide.

But now that we are adults and can provide our own shelter and food, we no longer have such a desperate need to please authority figures. However, some of us have recreated the dynamics of our original families in our personal lives and in our work places. And so the need to be phony, to get approval and promotions, and even to keep our jobs, seems as compelling as ever.

But the truth is, we can find people who approve of the real us as easily as we can find those who would try to smash us down. We are simply in the habit of trying to please others (many of whom cannot be pleased under any conditions, which guarantees that the energy of the people-pleasers will continue coming their way) and so we find those people with whom we can act out that scenario.

Once we begin to discover the truth about the world

and ourselves, we will make choices that contribute to our physical, spiritual, mental and emotional well-being. We were not brought to this Earth to be miserable. We are not intrinsically sinful. That untruth is promoted to keep in business those who would be our saviors. We have fallen for some powerful lies based on other people's agendas.

For us to discover our true selves, and to have full-blown bowel movements, we must turn away from the lies that hurt us and turn inward to the truth of our beings.

And as with learning anything new, it takes time to discover the inner self. But what could be a better investment of time? The world needs our true selves. We need our true selves. Our children and dogs and mates and employees and employers need our true selves.

What are the techniques for discovering the truth? Just the intent to do so is the most powerful factor. After that is established, anything creative will help us figure it out.

Many of us try abstract painting, making collages, writing poetry, playing music, making jewelry, or even cooking (provided, of course, that we don't eat to escape from ourselves). In creative activity, we are challenged to make decisions and choices that are not based on anyone's rules, but on our own unique perspective. Do I put the blue paint here or the red paint? Does the orange bead go here or there? And would basil or rosemary be most delicious in this dish?

Each time we go inside and listen to the still, small voice that urges us to make a certain decision, we are honoring our true selves, the one who has been lying in wait since childhood.

Sure, it's a lifelong process to discover one's self. But what else are we going to do in the meantime? Continue blotting out the truth of our beings? I don't think so.

Write On

Write about the activities you have done in life which you sensed tapped into your deepest, creative self. Write about the activities which seemed to touch you in a very deep way.

My list would include writing poetry and making collages. Try to be specific about what exactly happens inside you when you do these things. In collage, I get to activate and enjoy what I call my "Yes/No" facility. For each piece of paper I am thinking of adding to my collage, I get a feeling inside that says yes, put it here, or no, don't put it here. My exercise is to trust the feeling and place or not place the item in my artwork. I also rely on this hard-to-describe feeling when deciding whether or not the piece is finished. People have often asked me how I know when a piece is finished. It all hinges on that inner knowledge, and in obeying it. The finished artworks are not my primary focus in this exercise, although they have given me and others much enjoyment, but my focus is on the process.

As an aside, when I practice this Yes/No exercise, I also find myself getting more open sexually. In fact, when I find myself shutting down sexually, I can usually get my Eros energized with an hour or so of collage work.

Affirmation of Truth:

My true inner self is exciting and sexy and dynamic and unpredictable and has never been known on this planet before nor will it be known after I leave. I honor this self and express it.

Chapter 11

Letting Darkness Be Darkness

I am ashamed of these tears. And yet
At the extreme of my misfortune
I am ashamed not to shed them.

—*Euripides*

Let your tears come. Let them water your soul.

—*Eileen Mayhew*

My grief was too deeply rooted to be cured with words.

—*Orinda*

For women, the door into feelings is pain. For men, the door is grief.

—*Robert Bly*

To spare oneself from grief at all cost can be achieved only at the price of a total detachment, which excludes the ability to experience happiness.

—Erich Fromm

We are healed of suffering only by experiencing it to the full.

—Marcel Proust

Those who do not know how to weep with their whole heart don't know how to laugh either.

—Golda Meir

You must travel the river, live on it, follow it when there is morning light, and follow it when there is nothing but dark and the banks have blurred into shadows.

—Wil Haygood

When the friendly lights go out, there is a light by which the heart sees.

—Olga Rosmanith

The height of wisdom is to take things as they are. . . to endure what we cannot evade.

—Montaigne

If you can't fight and you can't flee, flow.

—Robert Eliot

One often learns more from ten days of agony than from ten years of contentment.

—Merle Shain

What wound did ever heal but by degrees?

—William Shakespeare

There is something infinitely healing in the repeated refrains of nature—the assurance that dawn comes after night, and spring after the winter.

—Rachel Carson

When it gets dark enough, you can see the stars.

—Lee Salk

Strange feelings. . . . Just a sort of unexplained sadness that comes each afternoon when the new day is gone forever and there's nothing ahead but increasing darkness.

—Robert Pirsig

It is not often given in a noisy world to come to the places of great grief and silence.

—Sarah Orne Jewett

There are occasions where it is undoubtedly better to incur loss than to make gain.

—Plautus

We lop away, that bearing boughs may live.

—William Shakespeare

A depressing and difficult passage has prefaced every new page I have turned in life.

—Charlotte Bronte

Oh, what we won't do to get out of feeling our emotional pain! Ouch! We just won't have it. There's no reason for pain when we have the handy opiates of excess sugar, food, drugs, alcohol, television, shopping, sex and exercise (I'd like to have this last problem for just a day or a week!).The list goes on. Our whole culture is so geared to getting rid of the pain that we have no awareness of any alternative—like simply feeling the pain, much less honoring it and appreciating it.

Now this can get tricky. Especially if we are consciously following a spiritual path, we might decide that pain is not spiritual and so we refuse to participate in it. We say we will "turn it over" to our higher powers. We walk around with serene-looking half smiles on our lips, acting like everything is just so wonderful, so peaceful. I know one woman who wore a flowing white gown to her husband's funeral. Where is the balance in that? I just hope she was wearing black undergarments.

But this attempt to look serene leaves us feeling empty. For when we try to shut down one part of ourselves, our grief, we shut down much more than that. Sometimes we shut down all of ourselves. And when we shut down legitimate pain, refusing to allow it to flow through us, our bodies reflect that perfectly and we are once more constipated, plugged up, polluted. Obviously, we can't have that. We are meant to live in the flow of the universe and let the universe flow through us.

The surprising solution to this problem is to allow the feelings of pain happen, observe them, and let them pass. Think of it like a river. The river that passes by us this moment is a totally different river from the one that passes by in the next moment. Different molecules. Our pain is like that. It flows through us like a river, sometimes like white water and sometimes like a glacier, or so it seems. But eventually the pain is played out and it is over, provided we don't keep trying to recreate it. This is a glorious, cleansing process, like a forest fire through overly dense brush. Getting excited and trying to find a way to put it out is natural. But if we can remember the principle of flow, we can actually sink down into the pain, experience it, and let it run its course.

The fear is that the emotional pain will never end, that this pain I have now—this grief or this shame or this sorrow or this anguish—is now a permanent fixture in my life and unless I do something *right now* I will be overcome now and forevermore. This is not true. Most of us have known only two ways to deal with pain: deny it or be overcome by it. But we can choose a middle path, which is to notice it the pain, feel the pain, observe the pain, and not be destroyed by it. We are not our pain. We are what is feeling the pain, what is observing the pain.

Actually, the pain is not the problem. It's our reaction to it, our fight of it. The amount of psychic energy it takes to hold back the truth is enormous. We are sickened and exhausted by our fight, often investing many, many more times the energy into stopping a pain than it would take to just feel it. Scott Peck says in "The Road Less Traveled" that mental illness comes from the attempt to block legitimate pain.

Perhaps only by experience can many of us really believe this principle of being with our pain. Only by refraining from overeating or drinking alcohol or earning yet another college degree or whatever during a time of painful feelings can we observe the flow of them—the beginning, the middle and then end of them. "Here comes a feeling," we might say when a tragedy occurs where intense feelings would be a normal experience. "Here it is," we could say in the thick of it. "There it goes," we can say when the process is complete. And it does get completed.

I just had the experience of laughing in my therapist's office at the antics of a rude, self-centered family member who has caused me so much pain in my life. Because I refuse to see this person, I am not continually being hurt. And, at the same time, the pain of the childhood abuse has finally been felt, I think. There is no more pain, at this moment anyway. A recent phone call from this person was hysterical in its attempts to make me feel guilty, to control my energy. I got off the phone as soon as possible, because it was not pleasant. But afterward, I found the whole thing so funny. I'll tell you, I never expected to stop sobbing about the childhood abuse. And yet here I am, giggling in the present over these continuing antics.

Life is tremendous, moving, emotional, messy. Let's not deny that, let's not try to be stick figures. We were born human so we could have human experiences. Painful feelings are part of that. Our feelings are valuable sources of information for us. When we feel shame, it's often because we have acted in an unwholesome manner. When we feel grief, it's a barometer of how much we have lost, of how deeply we have loved. Is that so bad?

Let us honor ourselves, our processes. Let us not spend thousands of dollars on chemicals designed to take us away from ourselves. If we do, our brilliant bodies will continue to get sicker and sicker, trying desperately to alert us that something is terribly wrong. And then we will need more medicines, more laxatives, more doctors, more people getting rich off our malady.

We can have a new theology. We can truly believe that everything that happens to us is for our benefit. Everything. If we would but look for the lesson, instead of fighting the pain, we will get the lessons we need. We are not mistaken. We are not wrong. Our experiences are not punishments. We are loved in our totality by this universe that wants us to be here. We are deeply welcome here.

Write On:

Close your eyes and remember a time of great pain for you. Perhaps it was the death of a parent or of a child or of a pet. Perhaps it was during incest therapy, or in the pits of alcoholism or compulsive overeating or spending. Remember how it felt to be in that dark, hopeless place. Write about it. Put down in words all you. remember. Make it real. Don't be alarmed if a few more or a lot more tears come out. Let it happen.

When you have honored the experience on paper, or in an artwork, or in a poem, remember how you came out of the darkness, how you talked with people, with friends and family and counselors. Recall how you once felt like life had no meaning, and recall a time past that when life was once again joyful. Think about the whole thing as one experience—before pain, during pain, after pain.

We have all lived through so much pain, starting with our own birth. If we can remember how we have already lived through and survived pain, then we can have more faith next time that we will endure. Why grow old, as we are doing, unless we can learn the lesson of endurance? We will survive.

Affirmation of Truth:

I have survived pain in the past and I will survive any pain that comes to me in the future. Even in darkness, I am a survivor. I do not fight the darkness.

Chapter 12

Losing Our Denial of Death

Death, when it approaches, ought not to take one by surprise. It should be part of the full expectancy of life.

—*Muriel Spark*

Whoever is interested in life is particularly interested in death.

—*Thomas Mann*

A dying (person) needs to die as a sleepy (person) needs to sleep, and there comes a time when it is wrong, as well as useless, to resist.

—*Stewart Alsop*

The world is impermanent. One should constantly remember death.

—*Sri Ramakrishna*

Birth is not one act; it is a process. The aim of life is to be fully born, though its tragedy is that most of us die before we are thus born. To live is to be born every minute. Death occurs when birth stops.

—Erich Fromm

The Buddhist Sutra of Mindfulness speaks about the meditation on the corpse: meditate on the decomposition of the body, how the body bloats and turns violet, how it is eaten by worms until only bits of blood and flesh still cling to the bones, meditate up to the point where only white bones remain, which in turn are slowly worn away and turn into dust. Meditate like that, knowing that your own body will undergo the same process. Meditate on the corpse until you are calm and at peace, until your mind and heart are light and tranquil and a smile appears on your face. Thus, by overcoming revulsion and fear, life will be seen as infinitely precious, every second of it worth living.

—Thich Nhat Hanh

Human beings are afraid of dying. They are always running after something: money, honor, pleasure. But if you had to die now, what would you want?

—Taisen Deshimaru

You don't get to choose how you're going to die, or when. You can only decide how you're going to live. Now.

—Joan Baez

When you cease to make a contribution, you begin to die.

—Eleanor Roosevelt

When we are no longer children, we are already dead.

—Konstantin Brancust

Later. I'm still young. I'll think of spiritual things when I'm older. On my deathbed.

—Garrison Keillor

To live fully one must risk death and accept its ultimate decision.

—Judd Mamor

Granted that I must die, how shall I live?

—Michael Novak

All (people) should strive to learn before they die what they are running from, and to, and why.

—James Thurber

I do not want to die. . . until I have faithfully made the most of my talent and cultivated the seed that was placed in me until the last small twig has grown.

—Kathe Kolwitz

And it isn't the thing you do, dear,
It's the thing you leave undone
Which gives you a bit of a heartache
At the setting of the sun.

—Margaret Sangster

It is frightful not to live.

—Victor Hugo

I postpone death by living, by suffering, by error, by risking, by giving, by losing.

—Anais Nin

Everything has an end.

—Masai saying

Death is not failure. Let's hear that again. Death is not failure. It is not punishment. It is not aberration. It is as fully a part of a human life as is being born. So far, no human has gotten one without the other. And yet we live in a culture that is terrified and repulsed by death. It reminds me of the way we are all repulsed by feces, by the very mention of bowel movements. Both are natural and as much a part of us as our smiles or our capacities to love.

To deny or dread that which is one hundred percent certain to happen is surely the way to deep misery. There is no benefit to us in all this denial. It will not make death go away if we pretend it is not coming. It's like the waves in the ocean. Try standing on the beach and dread the waves. Try to hate them. Fear them. Deny them. What happens? The waves continue to break upon the shore. Why waste precious life energy on denying death when it will come just the same?

The best reason to come to some acceptance about our deaths is to have better lives now, free from the sickness and constipation that denial brings. To fully live, we need to honor that part of our life that will surely come to us—our own death. Our dying itself can be a very sacred time. The hospice movement, where people with terminal illness are encouraged to die at home with loved one, is not only about death. It is about living one's last, precious days to the fullest.

Just because we live in a death-denying society does not mean that we must do likewise, digging in our heels to avoid (always unsuccessfully) an experience our creator obviously wants for us. We can fill in the gaps in our understanding and become more conscious and accepting of our own death. We can attend death-and-dying workshops, be a hospice volunteer, read books about dying with dignity.

One reason we are so afraid to die is because so many of us have not lived our true lives. As children, we (our authentic selves) were not wanted by our parents. As Alice Miller says in her book, "The Drama of the Gifted Child," our parents wanted someone else. They wanted their vision of who we should be to be fulfilled. And so to survive, many of us took on fake personalities that conformed to our parents' desires. And maybe those pleasing facades have even brought us fame and fortune. But with such an estrangement from our personal truths, our being knows that something very important is not happening in this lifetime. And decades of a fake personality, even if it is considered successful by society's standards, will not give us the feeling of completion that we would like to have at the end of our lives. Pleasing others will not give us peace.

We can now respect ourselves for surviving, for doing what we had to do, and begin the journey of reclaiming our true selves. For it is only by fully becoming our own authentic selves that we feel we have done what we were brought to this Earth to do. Surely just surviving, just getting by, is not why we are here. It is not enough for the dignified likes of us, for those of us desperate to be whole and happy.

Meditate on just how complex it is to bring a human being to this planet, to find caretakers for that person, to feed, clothe, house and love that person. And that person will need a job and hobbies and relationships and experiences and challenges and problems and solutions. Some great energy has gone to a lot of trouble to bring us here and make a space for us. Why are we here? Have we let our unique gifts be developed into something that can nurture the Earth and its people? If not, if we continue to hold back the best of who we are, our constipation and fear of death will remain.

As Philip Doddridge said: "Let us live while we live." And later, we can die in fullness and without regret.

Write On:

Think for a moment on the end of your life. Imagine you have lived a full life and it is time to go. What would you like to feel like at that time? Write about what you would like to have accomplished by your last day. What kind of person would you like to be? With what qualities? I would like to be very powerful and kind by the end of my lifetime, to have written movies and/or books that made people feel stronger and more blessed.

Write about your memorial service. Write about how you want it arranged, what people might say. For me, I would like people to come to a microphone and say how they knew me, what knowing me meant to them, how what I was here made the world a better place.

If we focus on our own deaths, we can live fully now.

Affirmation of Truth:

I will be on this Earth for a limited time, and I will make the most of these blessed days.

V

Letting Life Flow

Zen teaches us to discover the transcendental core of our own selves in an immediate and practical sense, to "taste" divine Being in the here-and-now.

—Karlfried Graf Durkheim

Chapter 13

Giving From an Overflowing Cup

The greatest gift we can give one another is rapt attention to another's existence.

—***Sue Atchley Ebaugh***

The only gift is a portion of myself.

—***Ralph Waldo Emerson***

On action alone be thy interest, never on its fruits.

—***Bhagavad Gita***

It's not what we see and touch or that which others do for us which makes us happy; it is that which we think and feel and do, first for the other fellow and then for ourselves.

—***Helen Keller***

If I can stop one heart from breaking,
I shall not live in vain;
If I can ease one life the aching,
Or cool one pain,
Or help one fainting robin
Into (its) nest again,
I shall not live in vain.

—Emily Dickinson

I came to understand that it was all right to do things for people as long as I did it for the sake of doing it. . . , the value being more in the act than in the result.

—Joanna Field

Service. A beautiful word fallen upon hard times.

—Claude McKay

and if ever i touched a life i hope that life knows that i know that touching was and still is and always will be the true revolution

—Nikki Giovanni

Cast thy bread upon the waters; for thou shalt find it after many days.

—Ecclesiastes 11:1

For the whole law is fulfilled in one word, "You shall love your neighbor as yourself."

—Galatians 5:14

Keep your hands open, and all the sands of the desert can pass through them. Close them, and all you can feel is a bit of grit.

—Taisen Deshimaru

There should be less talk; a preaching point is not a meeting point. What do you do then? Take a broom and clean someone's house. That will say enough.

—Mother Teresa

Every year I live I am more convinced that the waste of life lies in the love we have not given, the powers we have not used. . . .

—Mary Cholomondeley

Every truth we see is one to give to the world, not to keep to ourselves alone.

—Elizabeth Cady Stanton

Complete possession is proved only by giving. All you are unable to give possesses you.

—Andre Gide

To receive everything, one must open one's hands and give.

—Taisen Deshimaru

Giving is the greatest gift of the mind.

—Helen Keller

Let us not be satisfied with just giving money; money is not enough. The poor need our hands to serve them. They need our hearts to love them.

—Mother Teresa

As babies, the first things of physical substance we each had to give the world were our glorious bowel movements. And surely we were proud of what we had brought forth, this early intimate present, this deepest of all gifts.

But it didn't take us long to realize that our gift was not valued by others. We saw adults holding their noses, making negative sounds and removing the offending parcel as soon as possible. For some of us, holding back our gift seemed the proper thing to do.

Later—or sooner—we learned to hold back our bowel movements until certain moments when it was acceptable to let go. Then, we got praise, love and kisses. But if we let go before or after that moment, the punishment was shaming and even physical violence. Ah, how complicated our first gift had become!

For many of us, our held-in bowel movements were just the beginning of a totally held-in person. We might have despised ourselves and believed that anything that came out of us was shameful and a pollution to the Earth. Perhaps we felt our greatest job was to hold back the filth and evil that lurked inside. And many of us did a pretty good job of that. I was a master.

But, of course, this could not continue. Our true selves—which are awesome combinations of power and beauty—are not content to stay hidden and be denied. Even with all our consciousness-blotting methods (overindulgence in drugs, food, alcohol, masturbation, TV), those selves will not allow us to rest. Like persistent dogs scratching at the door, our souls will not give up. And so our false selves are giving up the show and we have started the long journey of surrendering to who we truly are.

For us, recovery is a process of elimination. We have to let go of all the lies about ourselves that we had taken for the truth—mainly that we are inherently flawed. Once we root out the lies, perhaps with the help of loving friends and professionals, we are left more or less with ourselves as we were at birth. We have much talent, but none of the adult discipline that every artist needs. And we are all artists; our life is our greatest artwork. Slowly we develop the muscles we need to express our art in writing, painting, gardening, child rearing, love-making—in life.

And there's more good news. After we recover our true selves, something perhaps quite unexpected begins to happen. We begin to be intensely interested in the well-being of others. Not a co-dependent interest—where I take care of your so that you will take care of me—but a true and deep welling up of ourselves and an overflowing of our love for others. It seems that only by meeting our true selves are we ready to and capable of meeting others.

I feel sad when I hear disparaging remarks made about the self-help movement that has swept across our society. Some see it as self-centered stinginess instead of what it really is—building the foundation for a more loving world. People who are afraid of knowing their true selves will sometimes degrade those who go inside for the truth. So be it. We must press ahead with our mission for spiritual and physical health.

We cannot give from a substanceless cup, that is, from a cup full of falseness, full of pretense. The only way we can make our contribution to the good of the world—which I am convinced we desperately want to do—is to heal ourselves from the inside out. When we do, our talents will flow and our love will flow. And healthy bowel movements will flow as well.

Write On:

Think back to early childhood, to times when you had a deep, overpowering desire to help the world around you. Perhaps you nursed an injured bird or pet back to health. Maybe you felt sorry for a poor family and helped their children have fun. Before we lost our true selves into hiding, we were naturally compassionate. Write about this and remember vividly how you felt then.

Affirmation of Truth:

As I allow my authentic self to grow and thrive, I will naturally want to share my merits with the world.

Chapter 14

Personal Growth Is Our Greatest Gift

Love is above all, the gift of oneself.

—Jean Anouilh

If you have knowledge, let others light their candles at it.

—Margaret Fuller

But where was I to start? The world is so vast, I shall start with the country I know best, my own. But my country is so very large. I had better start with my town. But my town, too, is large. I had better start with my street. No, my home. No, my family. Never mind, I shall start with myself.

—Elie Wiesel

If a (person) wants to be of the greatest possible value to (one's) fellow-creatures, let (one) begin the long, solitary task of perfecting (oneself).

—Robertson Davies

There's only one corner of the universe that you can be certain of improving and that's your own self.

—Aldous Huxley

Transformation begins on an individual level and moves out into the world.

—Shakti Gawain

How shall we expect charity toward others, when we are uncharitable to ourselves?

—Sir Thomas Browne

Without health and courage we cannot face the present or the germ of the future in the present, and we take refuge in evasion.

—Cyril Connolly

When health is absent, wisdom cannot reveal itself, art cannot manifest, strength cannot fight, wealth becomes useless, and intelligence cannot be applied.

—Herophilus

Let everyone sweep in front of his or her own door, and the whole world will be clean.

—Goethe

So you want to be a positive influence in the world? First, get your own life in order.

—John Heider

So familiar—and so sad—are those who try so hard to help others that they neglect their own bodies, families and lives. This could be true for some of us who are predisposed to constipation. Since being clogged up and in pain could be interpreted as a divinely ordained punishment, it may seem as though helping others will give us the "brownie points" we need to gain favor with God and the universe. Alas, as many of us have discovered, this doesn't work. Ironically, the way we can be of most use to our fellow human beings is to be in fit mental, emotional, physical, and spiritual condition.

While many regularly nourish their souls in nature and at retreat centers, there are also those who feel guilty taking that luxury time when 40,000 children are starving to death on this planet every day. That feeling is understandable. But it's not useful. For instance, Mother Teresa, our symbol for selfless giving, spends several hours in the morning in prayer. Imagine how many more dying people she could hold in those hours, and yet she spends them in communion with her God. She explains our need for spiritual nourishment: "To keep a lamp burning, we have to keep putting oil in it."

Actually, to think that we can give to others constantly and without refueling is a very egotistic proposition. It takes a true humility, often developed through painful lessons, to admit that we are not bottomless wells of energy and love. Even the most generous of us get weary and need rest.

As we come to understand our own processes, we may see that our capacities to give love are like the ocean: we have high tides and low tides. We have a rhythm. After dismantling the lie that we are inherently worthless, we learn to trust ourselves. When we feel depleted, we nurture ourselves, knowing that we will eventually feel like giving once again.

As Elisabeth Kübler-Ross writes: "The ultimate lesson all of us have to learn is unconditional love, which includes not only others but ourselves as well."

Write On:

Write about the times when you were supremely helpful to another human being. Think of times when you were really of service, not co-dependently so. Write about your feelings of strength and health.

Now write about the ways you nurture your mental, physical, emotional and spiritual health. Do you give yourself the care you need?

Affirmation of Truth:

As I come into my own full, robust health, I have the deep desire to be of service. When I am depleted of health, I pause and refresh myself, until I am ready to serve again.

Chapter 15

Creativity Springs From Our Authentic Selves

Use what talents you have; the woods would have little music if no birds sang their song except those who sang best.

—*Rev. Oliver G. Wilson*

Art and poetry have always been altering our ways of sensing and feeling—that is to say, altering the human body.

—*Norman O. Brown*

It is the creative potential itself in human beings that is in the image of God.

—*Mary Daly*

By their fruits you shall know them.

—***Jesus***

If our reliance is upon anything but our own understanding of Truth, our work will cease to be fruitful.

—***Emmet Fox***

The oppressed must realize that they are fighting not merely for freedom from hunger, but for. . . freedom to create and to construct, to wonder and to venture.

—***Paulo Freire***

Life is painting a picture, not doing a sum.

—***Oliver Wendell Holmes Jr.***

We ordinary people must forge our own beauty. We must set fire to the grayness of our labor with the art of our own lives. In this kind of creation, every day becomes pure enjoyment.

—***Kenji Miyazawa***

I believe that true identity is found. . . in creative activity springing forth from within. It is found, paradoxically, when one loses oneself. Woman can best re-find herself by losing herself in some kind of creative activity of her own.

—***Anne Morrow Lindbergh***

Art is the basic form of meditation. . . . With art as meditation, creation as blessing is rediscovered and our trust in letting go is affirmed.

—***Matthew Fox***

Every totalitarian regime is frightened by the artist.

—***Walter Brueggemann***

What good is it to me if Mary gave birth to the son of God fourteen hundred years ago and I do not also give birth to the son of God in my time and in my culture?
—Meister Eckhart

It's not surprising that so many of us don't consider ourselves artists. A sampling of society's mind set finds a lot of negative images connected with artists: insane, poor, out of touch with the world, tending toward suicide. In this patriarchal world, based on the domination of some over others (which we have lived under for the past 5,000 years of our 300,000 years of human history, and which seems to be coming to an end), art is not encouraged, except for the elite, privileged few. For as Rollo May said in his book, "Courage to Create," "Artists are generally soft-spoken persons who are concerned with their inner visions and images. But this is precisely what makes them feared by any coercive society. For they are the bearers of the human being's age-old capacity to be insurgent."

The truth is, everyone who is open to her or his inner self has artistic visions and images. However, governments and advertisers have a big stake in keeping us dependent on them and their images in order for them to be rich and powerful to make up for their own lack of true self-awareness. The result is powerful propaganda leveled against our artistic energy. And we obey like dutiful children, holding ourselves back, even though we don't even know what it is we are holding back.

All this holding back is manifested in our bodies, which never lie. We end up constipated, unable to let go of our art, which has been deemed unacceptable, unwanted, unneeded. But finally we have come to a crossroads. Do we live sickly half lives or do we take a chance on letting the unknown come forth? If you are reading this book of encouragement, you must have chosen the latter path.

Think back on your early life if you can, before you were stifled. What did you really, really love to do? Finger painting? Playing with your dog? Making up stories? We are born with deep love for something, for many things. Many of us will deny that we have any creative passion at all. But with some probing and thought, the truth comes out. Most of us have felt deep, almost overwhelming passion in our early lives, but learned to shut that down for pure survival purposes.

OK, so we survived. Congratulations to us all. But we're not three years old anymore. Our survival doesn't depend on pleasing Mommy and Daddy. Part of the trouble is that we have not made the connection that what we love to do is indeed our life work. We've been fed the lie that work is hard and life is miserable. It can be, but only if we believe that. If we adopt a new way of thinking, where we believe the universe loves us and needs us and wants us to be fulfilled, we will naturally start seeing our passions as our true work.

Do we love to create graphics on our computer? Then why are we a carpenter? Do we love building with wood? Then why are we a graphic artist?

Are we fascinated with interpersonal relationships and want to help people work things out? Then why are we a telephone operator? Do we love making things? Then why are we watching TV? It's truly amazing how many of us have gone in the opposite direction of our hearts' desires. I spent many years working in fast-food restaurants—just the worst possible thing for a compulsive overeater!

Once we start trusting that our urges are divine, we will start listening to and following them instead of trying desperately to blot them out. We will have no peace anyway until we do what we have in us to do. Of course, following our hearts is going to be frightening at first, probably the most frightening thing we will ever do. This is putting our true selves out there, not some false mask. As Erica Jong writes:"And the trouble is, if you don't risk anything, you risk even more."

Instead of focusing on our fear of expressing ourselves, we can zero in on the excitement of it. Rollo May wrote: "We are living at a time when one age is dying and the new age is not yet born. . . . We are called upon to do something new, to confront a no-person's land, to push into a forest where there are not well-worn paths and from which no one has returned to guide us. . . . To live into the future means to leap into the unknown."

Once we have let go of the lie about our unworthiness, we begin to see that our artistic visions (as well as our bowel movements) are welcome—indeed are desperately needed—on this planet. We can start today to allow the truth of our beings to flow.

Write On:

Think back to a time when you were really creative. Maybe you were putting together a flower arrangement. Or maybe you were arranging a family reunion. Or maybe you were painting a chair. Make a list of those times you acted in ways that required a lot of creativity. How did you feel at those times? Sink down into those memories and remember just how it was for you.

Now, imagine that those times of sweet creativity were springing from your true self, the self that is hooked up to all the good energy of the universe. Take a few moments and wonder at being so connected to the creator of the universe.

Affirmation of Truth:

I am a co-creator with the creator of the universe. As I am fit and healthy, I create beauty in my world. I am hooked into the deep, blessed powers of the Earth.

Chapter 16

Living Fully in This Moment

The present moment is a powerful goddess.

—***Goethe***

Do what you can, with what you have, where you are.

—***Theodore Roosevelt***

We are here and it is now. Further than that all human knowledge is moonshine.

—***H. L. Mencken***

Perhaps this very instant is your time. . .your own, your peculiar, your promised and presaged moment, out of all moments forever.

—***Louise Bogan***

Do not set your eyes on things far off.

—***Phythian Odes***

This—the immediate, everyday, and present experience is IT, the entire and ultimate point for the existence of a universe.

—Alan Watts

If there is a sin against life, it consists perhaps not so much in despairing of life as in hoping for another life and in eluding the implacable grandeur of this life.

—Albert Camus

Our grand business is not to see what lies dimly at a distance, but to do what lies clearly at hand.

—Thomas Carlyle

I have come to believe in the "Sacrament of the Moment," which presupposes trust in the ultimate goodness of my creator.

—Ruth Casey

Every situation—nay, every moment—is of infinite worth; for it is the representation of a whole eternity.

—Goethe

Only in a hut built for the moment can one live without fear.

—Kamo no Chomei

The present time has one advantage over every other—it is our own.

—Charles Caleb Colton

Let me tell thee, time is a very precious gift of God; so precious that it's only given to us moment by moment.

—Amelia Barr

Life just is. You have to flow with it. Give yourself to the moment. Let it happen.

—Jerry Brown

One of the most tragic things I know about human nature is that all of us tend to put off living. We are all dreaming of some magical rose garden over the horizon—instead of enjoying the roses that are blooming outside our windows today.

—Dale Carnegie

When we pay attention, whatever we are doing—whether it be cooking, cleaning or making love—is transformed and becomes part of our spiritual path. We begin to notice details and textures that we never noticed before; everyday life becomes clearer, sharper, and at the same time more spacious.

—Rick Fields

Why are some of us so unhappy? So dissatisfied? So resentful? Why do we feel so ripped off, like we never got our share of the world's blessings? Maybe it's because we spend our energy remembering/regretting the past or fantasizing about/fearing the future. Of course we're tired, lost and frightened. Of course we're constipated.

That feeling of lack leads to petty thievery and white lies, which leads to shame and more negativity. Some of us have the attitude written about by Chuck C., a sober member of Alcoholics Anonymous, in "A New Pair of Glasses." He once believed that he "had to lie, cheat and steal to eke a miserable existence out of an unfriendly universe." But this attitude is based on a lie—the big lie that many people in our society want us to embrace—the lie that we're not OK and there's not enough to go around and that we need some product or service or leadership in order to get OK.

Now, there's nothing inherently wrong with people trying to sell us their goods. That's their job. But it is incumbent upon each one of us to find and champion our own truth within ourselves. To look to others for our truth is a mistake and leads to a fake, unsatisfactory life. It causes our bodies to seize up in fear. It causes us to trash today and to look ahead to some future point where things will finally be right. Or it causes us to wish for the past, when things were better. That leaves us with a today that is not worth sneezing at.

But the truth is that, for each of us, we live in the most perfect time ever. How could it be otherwise? Are we to be so egotistical to think that we know better than the creator? That the creator was mistaken in bringing us here now? I don't think so. We are all here for our ultimate good and everything we need for our soul's development is in our lives right at this moment.

Indeed, today is the one single chance we have in which to live out our lives. After all, yesterday's history and tomorrow's a mystery. Both of these times are valuable in their own ways, but they are not where the real juice of our lives lie, where we make our art, where we love our children, where we hug our dogs, where we make love, where we have our wondrous bowel moments. Trying to live out-of-touch with the present time is a sure way to confuse and abandon the body, which only functions in this moment.

One value in practicing appreciation of the present moment is that we can fully glory in the exquisite feeling of a full bowel moment. Our creator made us to enjoy our bodies, our minds, our emotions and our lives. If we are not hooked in with that essential birthright, that joy, we need to claim it and do whatever is necessary to have it. In meditation, it is a matter of eliminating the lies, the nonessential, the unnecessary.

If we would be awake in this moment, we might very well have an experience like Franz Kafka talks about when he says: "The world will freely offer itself to you to be unmasked, it has no choice, it will roll in ecstasy at your feet."

But the world only rolls in this very moment. As long as we're going to be here anyway, we might as well be awake.

Write On:

Take a moment and notice your surroundings. Now write about everything you can think of that is around you. I would write of my computer, the beautiful purple color on my monitor screen, the cool evening air touching the back of my arms, the sound of my partner tapping away at his computer, the sensation of my legs on the chair, the feeling of my feet on the floor, the slight tension between my eyes, the sounds of traffic outside my office door. And there is so much more.

Write about your very own moment, right here and now. What do you see, hear, feel, sense, smell? Keep writing about your present moment until it seems there is nothing missing at all from this universe in which you find yourself.

Affirmation of Truth:

In this moment is my whole life. There is nothing to my life, in this moment, than what I find here and now. This, THIS, is my life.

VI

Letting Happiness Happen

Happiness is the meaning and the purpose of life, the whole aim and end of human existence.

—Aristotle

Chapter 17

Getting a Dog
(or a Pot-Bellied Pig)

To err is human, to forgive canine.

—***Anonymous***

You think dogs will not be in heaven? I tell you, they will be there long before any of us.

—***Robert Louis Stevenson***

So many get reformed through religion. I got reformed through dogs. I underwent menopause without taking even an aspirin, because I was so busy whelping puppies. Dogs saved my life. I recommend having four-legged animals to cure the mid-life crisis.

—***Lina Basquette***

Dogs laugh, but they laugh with their tails.

—Max Eastman

Never have I experienced a serenity and sweetness of disposition as with my Chocolate Lab.

—Mortimer B. Zuckerman

Dogs' lives are too short. Their only fault, really.

—Agnes Sligh Turnbull

There is no faith which has never yet been broken except that of a truly faithful dog.

—Konrad Lorenz

I think we are drawn to dogs because they are the uninhibited creatures we might be if we weren't certain we knew better. They fight for honor on the first challenge, make love with no moral restraint, and they do not for all their marvelous instincts appear to know about death. Being such wonderfully uncomplicated beings, they need us to do their worrying.

—George Bird Evans

Dogs love company. They put it first on their short list of needs.

—J.R. Ackerley

Histories are more full of examples of the fidelity of dogs than of friends.

—Alexander Pope

The alliance between dogs and humans is the oldest, most durable, and most complete alliance between two species in history.

—Jon Winokur

Ever consider what they must think of us? I mean, here we come back from a grocery store with the most amazing haul—chicken, pork, half a cow. They must think we're the greatest hunters on Earth!

—Anne Tyler

The small percentage of dogs that bite people is monumental proof that the dog is the most benign, forgiving creature on Earth.

—W.R. Koehler

Living with a dog is easy—like living with an idealist.

—H.L. Mencken

All knowledge, the totality of all questions and all answers, is contained in the dog.

—Franz Kafka

We're to listen to a dog until we discover what is needed instead of imposing ourselves in the name of training.

—The Monks of New Skete
"How to Be Your Dog's Best Friend"

To have full and miraculous natural bowel movement, it's best to be happy deep inside. For happiness massages the intestines, I am sure. We must always ask ourselves—and our higher power—just what will make our hearts sing, our bellies laugh. For this is the favored way of the universe. A grand eucalyptus tree that is planted in the right place is quietly shouting for joy toward the sky and deep into the ground. Likewise, we were created—and also given the ability—to find the right soil, the right amount of water, the proper light for us to thrive.

For some of us, a canine companion is part of the happiness recipe, part of what gets our innards vibrating with joy. Now if you don't like dogs at all and you really commune best with cats or llamas or pot-bellied pigs, that's great. Feel free to collect a few pot-bellied pig quotes, write your own chapter called "Getting a Pot-Bellied Pig," and tape it into this book.

Imagine having a dog like my Good Golly Ms. Molly, the Springer Spaniel that has been a role model to me in my daily quest for spectacular bowel movements. At first light, you awaken and open the door so Molly can go outside. Sometimes, a neighbor dog in our mountainous neighborhood scratches first, asking if Molly can play.

Once the dogs are gone on their morning run in the back country, you eat breakfast and get some tea brewing. As is your morning routine, you cherish your quiet time, perhaps before the family or house mates arise, reading books about the higher power of your choice while you sip hot brew. Later, after you get that deep, centered feeling, you dip into the stack of newspapers near your bed.

By this time, Molly and her pal or pals are back and burst joyfully into your morning scene. With her beautiful brown eyes shining and her white belly wet from the morning dew, Molly slurps into her water bowl with wild abandon, sticking her snout deep into the water and splashing it all over the floor. At the same time, her stub of a tail is wagging madly. She looks up at you with blazing eyes, rivers of water streaming from her soft mussel. The other dogs drink at the same time, but are invariably more refined, spilling nothing.

After Molly Dog has drunk or sloshed most of the water out of the bowl, she steps back and gives herself a complete shake, starting at her brown nose and ending with her little butt. Of course, water flies all over the room. That done, your little friends go outside to stretch out in the morning sunlight, and you get up and wipe up the mess.

Now, you've never been accused of being a patient person, but watching this morning scene causes you no resentment at all. Quite the opposite. Every moment watching these elated dogs fills you with unspeakable joy and sets your innards a-twittering. If you've every tried drugs, you realize they never gave you anything near the fantastic feeling that you get with these dogs.

It's not long after this scenario that you begin to feel the urge from the great bowel movement goddess in the sky, and eventually you head for the bathroom to have a truly spiritual experience.

Now this is not to say that you must get a dog in order to have your daily miracle. But find what causes your heart to swell—be is raising a child or playing the violin or knitting doll clothes—and give yourself those experiences.

Also, Molly Dog is a wise and wonderful Zen master. She knows how to let things happen, to take it easy and not try to run the universe. She is not tied up in knots worrying about all the hungry dogs in the world. She takes care of her responsibilities—barking away intruders, chasing lizards, licking people and other dogs, sleeping close to her human's legs—and she trusts the Earth to take care of the rest.

When Molly is feeling clogged up, she changes her diet a little, usually adding a little bit of grass to get things moving again. And she has wonderful bowel movements, usually during daily hikes in the mountains. Her human companion pauses respectfully while Molly eliminates her bowels, always praising her with "What a good dog you are, Molly!" when she is done. Molly runs past, laughing, modeling the way to enlightenment. I wish I could love being a human as much as Molly loves being a dog.

Write On:

What brings you deep joy? Write about what rings your chimes, and include the feelings you get when you are doing these things. If you aren't doing something lately that makes your heart sing for joy, remember when you did something you loved when you were younger. Perhaps it was ballet. Or making slingshots. Or maybe you really, really love relaxing in spring grasses.

Make a list of those things which make life so sweet for you. Are you doing your loves of life as much as you want? What holds you back? Figure out some way to do more of what you love. Write down your solutions and refer to them often.

Affirmation of Truth:

I make time for what brings me joy. The deepest energies of the universe want to engulf me with happiness. I accept.

Chapter 18

Enjoying the Mystery

God hugs you.
You are encircled by the arms
of the mystery of God.

—Hildegard of Bingen

Everything has its wonders, even darkness and silence.

—Helen Keller

The epitome of irrationality is the marvel of creation itself.

—Otto Rank

The most beautiful experience we can have is the mysterious.

—Albert Einstein

Penetrating so many secrets, we cease to believe in the unknowable. But there it sits nevertheless, calmly licking its chops.

—*H.L. Mencken*

To know what we do not understand is the beginning of wisdom.

—*Maha Sthavira Sangharakshita*

It is impossible to begin to learn that which one thinks one already knows.

—*Epicetus*

Clever people seem not to feel the natural pleasure of bewilderments, and are always answering questions when the chief relish of life is to go on asking them.

—*Frank Moore Colby*

Gardening is an active participation in the deepest mysteries of the universe.

—*Thomas Berry*

The highest point a (person) can attain is not knowledge, or Virtue, or Goodness, or Victory, but something even greater, more heroic and more despairing: Sacred Awe!

—*Nikos Kazantzakis*

Be patient toward all that is unsolved in your heart
And try to love the questions themselves.

—*Rainer Maria Rilke*

I was gratified to be able to answer promptly, and I did. I said I didn't know.

—*Mark Twain*

Nobody has all the answers. Knowing that you do not know everything is far wiser than thinking that you know a lot when you really don't. Phony expertise is neurotic. . . it is a relief to be able to say, "I don't know."

—***John Heider***

(S/he) that knew all things that learning ever writ
Knew only this—that (s/he) knew nothing yet.

—***Aphra Behn***

If we want to stay really constipated, we can keep thinking that we know everything, or that we *must* know everything. It's not the thought that gets us, it's the gut-wrenching fear. Since it is absolutely impossible to know everything, the perceived need to do the impossible can only lead to inner terror. For some, fear may lead to loose bowels. But for we who were chosen to have this disposition toward constipation, inner terror means tightness and constipation.

But we cannot afford to be tight inside. Not if we want to let our true selves flow. Not if we want to have spectacular bowel movements. Rather, we need to maintain a state of inner relaxation. And the only way we can do that is to let go of our need to know everything.

Of course, this takes a lot of faith. As a constipated teenager, I had a series of nightmares where my job was to count every grain of sand on the beach. And that was just for starters. The ultimate task in these nightmares was to count every single molecule in the universe. The cause of the nightmare was a waking life so far away from knowing my authentic self that it seemed like knowing everything else in the world was the way to salvation. If everything was known, there would be safety. Then I could understand the crazy things that were happening around me.

For many of us, there's a certain excitement in thinking we could know it all, if only we applied ourselves. But since that is impossible, another way of being must be found. That way is to try to know our true selves as deeply as possible, treat those selves with utmost reverence, and have faith that the rest of the world is under the loving direction of a wise creator.

As we might come to believe, there is a goddess, and we ain't it. Whew! Isn't it exhausting trying to run the universe? The sheer tension of our responsibility caused our innards to seize up like a motor without oil.

Once we let some other power take care of most of the world, we can afford to actually delight in what is unknown to us. How exciting life really is, not knowing what the day will bring. Of course, we would be bored beyond belief if we did know everything. Actually, it's kind of fun not knowing what our pet is thinking, what she is dreaming about as she kicks and growls in her sleep. Who has not looked up into the countless stars with awe and humility? (If you live in a city where the stars are not visible, get yourself out into the country as soon and as often as possible.)

And while you're there, or even while in the city, look closely at a plant. See its leaves reaching for the sun, its flowers opening to the morning. How does it do that? Why does it do that? Sometimes it seems that the easiest thing for the great spirit of the universe to do would be to create no universe at all. But here it is. As one mystic said, god lies groaning on a birthing table all day long, giving birth to the universe.

Why should we not be intoxicated with that image? These are the images that get the body working, that fill a self with joy and mystery. We can't let the jaded, constipated part of the world get us down. We can't take on the numbness of the masses, at least not if we want full and wondrous bowel movements. They—and blatant, shameless awe—are our birthright.

Write On:

Isn't it amazing how little we really know, and yet how well our lives can function? Create two columns. On one side, make a list of things that affect you tremendously, and yet which you know so little about. Write about electricity, for instance. How much do we know? Even the scientists don't know how it works. And sunlight. How does that happen. In the second column, write about how these things benefit your life. The electricity powers your computer, gives light to you night, toasts your bread. The sunlight brightens your morning, blooms your roses, warms your dog's fur.

Write about these things until you get a deep feeling that all is well with the universe, that things are very perfect, even if we don't know all the answers.

Affirmation of Truth:

The world, which I didn't create and which I don't understand, is in perfect order and is awesomely beautiful. That I don't have all the answers is perfectly OK. I revel in the deep mysteries of the universe.

Chapter 19

We Are Meant to Be Happy

Joy enters the room. It settles tentatively on the windowsill, waiting to see whether it will be welcome here.

—*Kim Chernin*

I finally figured out the only reason to be alive is to enjoy it.

—*Rita Mae Brown*

Living itself (is) a task of such immediacy, variety, beauty, and excitement that one is powerless to resist its wild embrace.

—*E.B. White*

Just to be is a blessing.
Just to live is holy.

—*Abraham Heschel*

Everyone is in the best seat.

—John Cage

We are God's work of art.

—Eph 2:10

Grace spreads widely and shows the greatly abundant hospitality of the royal Lordship in God's astonishing courtesy toward us.

—Julian of Norwich

I sat there listening with my whole being, and with my whole strength contemplating that mountain that I so dearly love. . . . Was there anyone in the world, at that moment, as happy as I?

—Colette Richard

Taking joy in life is a woman's best cosmetic.

—Rosalind Russell

If you always do what interests you, then at least one person is pleased.

—Advice to Katherine Hepburn from her mother

If the only prayer you say in your whole life is "thank you," that would suffice.

—Meister Eckhart

I, God, am your playmate! I will lead the child in you in wonderful ways for I have chosen you.

—Mechtild of Magdeburg

Simply to live is a wonderful privilege in itself. . . .

—Henry Wood

Living in harmony with the universe is living totally alive, full of vitality, joy, power, love, and abundance on every level.

—*Shakti Gawain*

All that is required to feel that here and now is happiness is a simple, frugal heart.

—*Nikos Kantantzakis*

Most people are as happy as they make up their minds to be.

—*Abraham Lincoln*

Exuberance is beauty.

—*William Blake*

There is only one success—to be able to spend your life in your own way.

—*Christopher Morley*

To wildly happy in these troubled times? And in this very moment? What a radical concept! Who around us could tolerate us? Better to strive to be rich, or busy, or respected, or successful in one's field. Those are goals we can all understand. After all, these goals have guidelines. Perhaps it's better to be constipated and hating ourselves. Then we need to buy products and services to "fix" ourselves, and others will be grateful to get our money.

But to be happy? What are the requirements? Who can lead us?

And therein lies the rub. The only authority on our happiness is us. There is no handy scale of accomplishments that gives us society's seal of success in personal happiness. It is something that we must search for inside our own souls and we must dare to say we are happy if we are. And to admit that we're unhappy if we're not.

As I write this book, I live in a converted Southern Pacific caboose in the wooded mountains above Santa Barbara, California. In some ways, it is a small, pitiable existence that many people would not tolerate. And while I am privileged to have lived in several large and beautiful homes, I have never been so content as I am now. From my desk, I often pause in my work and gaze down the length of the caboose, soaking in the satisfying vision of a rosewood floor, a worn red quilt, flowers blooming by the window. And the forest of oak trees outside! How can one person have so many oak leaves in her life?

And by the way, this is the kind of happiness that makes a life of letting go — complete with regular bowel movements — possible for us. For if this simple life contains so much beauty, why do we need to grasp desperately onto anything? Instead, we can let go at the appropriate time and know that happiness will fill in the empty spaces within.

But it's amazing how many people settle for quiet — or unquiet— desperation, living unhappy, unfulfilled lives. And these people, in their fear that things could never be different for them, will quickly tell you that you are happy enough, that, indeed, no one is very happy.

But don't believe it! Unabashed joy is our birthright — that is partly why we are here. What a shame if we came to Earth this time around and forgot to appreciate our generous gift. For too many years, poisoned by the images of television and advertising, we have postponed our happiness until we would somehow be rich and famous and our stomachs would be flat. But those things never came. Or they came and went. And so we kept waiting.

As one spiritual friend has said many times, "God wants you to be happy, joyous and free. That is your natural state."

This is true and our higher power can really help us in this quest to be happy today. One lesson that has illuminated this understanding involves the more than 250 articles about houses I have written for my local newspaper. The assignment involves each week going to a different house (one that is not for sale) and interviewing the owners or renters.

This assignment has led to estates that are worth $20 million, as well as to mobile homes and even studio apartments. The observation is that wealth is not the answer to inner happiness, that we can give ourselves permission to go ahead and be happy right here and now, no matter what. Of course, the habit of our minds is to mess with us. "How can you be happy in such a place?" our minds tell us. "How can you be happy single/married/with these kids/without kids? You're supposed to have so much more/less than this." But these flimsy lies are no match for the deep contentment that can grow inside us.

And this claim to happiness does not mean that pain and grief and sadness are denied. For to deny the painful emotions is to deny them all. And to hold in the truth is to be constipated in a serious way. Actually, it's possible to feel a kind of elation inside even during a dark night of the soul. But even that's not necessary. To feel our deep grieving is holy.

And the good news is, these hard times pass and we are left experiencing the natural joy of being alive on even a deeper level. Perhaps we put off our happiness because we haven't grieved the experiences that are demanding a legitimate expression of grief. Ironically, the way into happiness is by moving down into our grief, when that is appropriate. Often, the only way out is through.

Wonderful bowel movements are both a result of happiness and a reason for it. Surely our creator meant us to have health on all levels. As Joseph Newton said, "God did not make us to be eaten up by anxiety, but to walk erect, free, unafraid in a world where there is work to do, truth to seek, love to give and win."

Once we have grieved our undeniable losses, there

is really no reason to delay moving toward happiness. Ultimately, the idea is to notice what makes us happy, and to move toward that. And to pay close attention to what makes us chronically unhappy and to move away from that. Avoid those incidents, people and activities. It's so simple, but how many of us do it? How many of us can break the misery habit?

A recent chat with a mentally retarded man illuminates our dilemma. The man said he used to bus tables at a pizza joint, a job he really loved. But the new managers fired him three years ago and now he sweeps the floors of a local mall. He said the new job is very boring.

"What would you really like to do?" I asked him. He's obviously given it much thought already and said he would love to work in another pizza joint or, better yet, at a flower stand.

"Have you tried to get a new job?" I said.

But he quickly lapsed into a singsong voice, saying he just has to make the best of a bad thing and not make it worse.

"No," I said forcefully, surprising even myself. "You have got to do what makes you happy. You've got to make sure you get what you want out of life." He creased his brow and went back to his magazine.

When challenged to come out of our misery, so many of us crease our brows and get back to our diversions. We want to live within our abilities, we say. Not disappoint ourselves by reaching too high. But I'm sure you've seen what I've seen: Many of us are reaching way too low.

Yes, moving toward happiness is quite an enormous task. But it's not a selfish thing. The anguish level of the entire planet is lessened every time one of us comes closer to accepting and moving toward our natural joy.

And from our places of vibrant joy, we have the love and energy to share ourselves with others. That's why this book was written. From one person's center overflowing with joy, you are humbly offered these words of encouragement and love and deep respect for your struggle—for you journey into the light.

Write On:

Having reached the last chapter, you have no writing assignment! That is your reward. You are to sit back in your chair and think of the many reasons there are for you to be happy. Just to be alive is at the top of the list. Count your blessings, for they are many.

And don't forget to pet your dog.

Affirmation of Truth:

My natural state is to be happy, joyous and free.

Appendix A:

An Odyssey Through Constipation Hell

I am ill because my mind is in a rut and refuses to leave.

-Karen Girodino

It's the awareness, the full experience . . . of how you are stuck, that makes you recover.

- Frederick S. Perls

Every time you don't trust your yourself and don't follow your inner truth, you decrease your aliveness and your body will reflect this with a loss of vitality, numbness, pain, and eventually, physical disease.

- Shakti Gawain

We're only as sick as the secrets we keep.

- ***Sue Atchley Ebaugh***

This is the story of my twenty-year journey through the hell of constipation and of my eventual freedom from it. But the good news first: Most days of the month, I have such full, glorious bowel movements that I think I must qualify for an award of some kind. I want to find someone and say, "Look! Look what I did!" Of course, this would be expected from a two-year-old. But from a forty-year-old? Still, I am joyous. That emptying-out feeling is something I wouldn't trade for all the dieter's tea in Chino.

Let people without this chronic constipation problem call themselves lucky. I guess I was unlucky, if you want to put it that way. As long as I can remember, in my teens and early adulthood, I was constipated, clogged up, full of it. It was just a way of life to have a bloated stomach, horrible gas pains, toxic farts, pimples, and boils on my butt that sent me to the emergency room to get lanced. Didn't everybody? Of course no one else did, I thought, and that made it all the worse. Lots of people are constipated, but few talk about it.

Imagine of we spoke the truth:

> ***Joe:*** *'Morning Gail How ya doing?*
> ***Gail:*** *Not good, Joe. I was constipated yesterday and was hoping for a big dump this morning. But*

no luck. How about you?
Joe: *I'm doing pretty good. The broccoli I ate yesterday really did the trick. I had a major BM this morning and I'm ready for the day.*

No, I don't think we'll be hearing this kind of conversation soon. But what could be more important, more intimate, more vital to feeling good?

If I tried to write about this in a newspaper essay, my editor would reject it, calling my language scatological. I'll save you a trip to the dictionary and tell you that scatology has two meanings: 1) the study of excrement and, 2) interest in obscene matter. So we've got this big scatological problem and it's too obscene to talk about. We can either remain polite and polluted or we can start talking (at least to each other) and get detoxified.

Ever notice that if there's a commercial on TV for laxatives, it's a big sniggering deal. The shame! The filth! And what's the answer? A bevy of harsh chemicals that can force your unwilling body to put out.

The Great Laxative Experiments

Laxatives and I have a long and intimate history. I started out with the most common kinds, Correctol ("the gentle woman's laxative") and Ex-Lax, which must have been created for "real men." Ex-Lax was definitely the king of commercial laxatives for me. Boy, does it work. It got that stuff shooting out of me like a garden hose going at full blast. Of course, there was a price to pay for all this release. I got white bumps all over and my body hair stood straight up on end. I got unbelievably painful abdominal cramps, as well as cramps in my legs and feet that woke me up screaming in pain in the middle of the night. Plus, I was tired after a bout with laxatives, had a pasty film over my skin and was irritable.

And that was just the surface stuff. The truth—and I knew this all along—is that taking laxatives caused my bowels to lose their ability to move at all. So each time I took laxatives, I got more dependent on them. It's like heroin for the hemorrhoid set.

Generally, I took laxatives once every three days—and this went on for at least 10 years. What was my alternative? Never empty my bowels? I've known people who don't have a bowel movement for weeks at a time. That wasn't for me, thank you very much. I needed to empty out the poisons in my system. (Even today, many years since I've found it necessary to do all that, my body cringes at these memories.)

Now please don't think I swallowed those laxatives lightly. I fervently wished my body would just start working right. I remember one humiliating Sunday morning, my third day without a bowel movement, walking around Santa Barbara trying to get my bowels moving. Walking, walking, walking—up and down those beautiful streets, aware of each abdominal sensation that might signal the beginning of a coveted BM.

But that morning it just wasn't happening and, as I had so many times before, I finally surrendered to failure. As I waited for a liquor store to open to buy some Ex-Lax, I was filled with shame at how I spent my Sunday morning, seeking the Goddess at the porcelain altar. Of course, it would take a few hours for the chemicals to work, but I knew once I tool the little pills, I was on my way to heaven.

Actually, I learned about laxatives from a family member who also suffered from constipation. She always had a box of little pink pills in the medicine cabinet. And from another relative, I learned about the magical qualities of prunes. She also suffered from constipation and couldn't live a day without her prunes.

"Natural" Ways to Force an Unwilling Body

Other times in my life I tried other creative—even holistic—measures. For a while, I was convinced that bran was the answer to my problem. The new problem was that I was constantly bloated. My method was to mix about a cup of dry bran flakes with two cups of water, open my throat and pour it in. I did this before each meal. It was probably the equivalent of eating one large cardboard box per day. I recently met a man who was recovering from appendix cancer that his doctors said was caused by undigested bran. It could be true.

Later I refined my bran habit and discovered psyllium husks. In water, this powder turns into a gelatin-like substance that you have to drink before it globs forever onto the bottom of your glass. This is the active substance in a certain laxative powder that some doctors have convinced some women, and men, they must take every day for the rest of their lives. For me, it had the same debilitating side effects as laxatives and the fact that doctors recommended it did not impress my body.

Sometimes I got on a water kick and drank gallons of water every day. This usually worked pretty well. But who has time to urinate every 10 minutes? After one good bowel movement from the water treatment, I usually turned back to commercial laxatives.

Then I discovered dieter's tea at the health food store. Now this stuff sounds great. It's all natural—even organic—and it doesn't say anything on the box about constipation. So how could it be a laxative?

Still, it had the exact same effect on my body as the chemicals. The same pimples, the same cramps, the same boils. And the worst thing was, I never lost any weight.

For a brief time, I enjoyed colonics. This is where you pay someone $30 or more to put a tube up your anus, pump warm water into your colon and then let it drain out, taking waste materials with it. It's actually a wonderful experience. And addictive. One friend of mine hasn't had natural bowel movements for years and instead has a colonic every three days. There are probably people who have them even more often. But for me, with my budget, $30 was too much for a regular habit. And besides, it didn't give me what I truly wanted in all the world: full, natural bowel movements.

Finally I got a doctor involved. He decided that there wasn't enough of the right bacteria in my digestive system. Following his written orders, I got a douche bag with a long tube and a quart of kefir milk, which is thick with the good bacteria the body needs.

At home, I filled the bag with the milk and warm water, put the tube in my anus and let my colon fill up with milk, which I held in there for half an hour. Let me tell you, those were some uncomfortable half hours naked on the bottom of a cold bathtub with my butt sticking up in the air. I'm sure the doctor had a good heart about it (or maybe he was a vicious sadist), but the ordeal didn't solve my problem and left me feeling even more humiliated.

Now here's something that I've never told anyone in the world and I'm not sure you want to hear it now. One time I got so desperate that I took a metal coat hanger and tried to dig excrement out of my anus. I hope no one reading this book has ever degraded themselves in that way. I'm taking major desperation.

So this has been a long struggle for me. I wish someone would give me a Ph.D. in scatology for all the research I've done.

Actually, I got a little constipated the morning I

started working on this book. That happens when I am nervous or fearful or when it's just before my period. But once I got going on the manuscript, my bowels gave up their bounty in miraculous form. Just this morning, I wanted someone to witness my morning miracle. For me, constipation is much more than just a physical problem. It has direct connections with my emotional and spiritual life. And this is real message of this book.

A Bowel-Related Miracle

But for all the yucky times I've had with my stubborn bowels, I also had one bowel-related experience that changed my life. It happened soon after I had joined a spiritually based fellowship that advocates prayer and meditation to help deal with addictions. At that time, I didn't believe in prayer. I had tried it as a kid and it didn't work. But I was a meditator and most of the other people in the group were not, so I figured we were equal.

Now this all happened during the time I was in the insanity of my bowel management programs, where every bowel movement was the result of some drastic measure—laxatives, water, bran, etc.

And then a miracle happened. One day, for no apparent reason, I had a spontaneous and unpremeditated bowel movement. I was practically in tears with gratitude. Still sitting on the pot, I turned my face upward and said, "Thank you."

I didn't know who or what I was thanking, but I knew this miracle came from some power greater than myself. That was my first prayer in adulthood. Since then I heard a quote from Meister Eckhart, a fourteenth century mystic, who said, "If the only prayer you ever said is 'Thank you,' that would suffice." And today that is the extent of my prayers: "Thank you."

Of course, after my morning miracle on that stupendous day, I didn't leave it at that. The next morning I got into position, looked up, and said: "Please."

Appendix B:

A Way of Letting Bowels Move

Zen aims at freedom but its practice is disciplined.
—*Gary Snider*

Without discipline, there's no life at all.
—*Katharine Hepburn*

Diseases desperate grown
By desperate appliances are relieved
Or not at all
—*Shakespeare*

True wisdom consists in not departing from nature and in molding our conduct according to her laws and model.
—*Seneca*

The process of changing a lifestyle is more important than reaching a goal or measuring a performance.

—Theodore Isaac Rubin

The body is the soul's house. Shouldn't we therefore take care of our house so that it doesn't fall into ruin?

—Philo Judaeus

I never suspected that I would have to learn how to live —that there were specific disciplines and ways of seeing the world that I had to master before I could awaken to a simple, happy, uncomplicated life.

—Dan Millman

In nature there are neither rewards nor punishments. There are consequences.

—Robert G. Ingersoll

I learned to listen to my body with an inner concentration like meditation, to get guidance as to when to exercise and when to rest. I learned that healing and cure are active processes in which I myself needed to participate.

—Rollo May

How much bondage and suffering a woman escapes when she takes the liberty of being her own physician of both body and soul.

—Elizabeth Cady Stanton

The message is, "It's okay if you mess up. You should give yourself a break."

—Billy Joel

Some people regard discipline as a chore. For me, it is a kind of order that sets me free to fly.

—Julie Andrews

It is a matter first of beginning—and then following through.

—Richard Evans

We need the courage to start and continue what we should do, and courage to stop what we shouldn't do.

—Richard Evans

The only true way of bringing about anything is by the Practice of the Presence of God. This is the only way in which permanent results can be obtained. Temporary alterations in conditions may be achieved by will power, but they are only temporary, and sooner or later anything that seems to have been accomplished in this way will disappear again, leaving everything worse than it was before.

—Emmet Fox

The preservation of health is duty. Few seem conscious that there is such a thing a physical morality.

—Herbert Spencer

What sort of God would it be, who only pushed from without?

—Goethe

(Important note: The following "formula for success" is my own story. It may have no bearing on your life and your body whatsoever. On the other hand, something you read here may strike within you a chord of recognition. My suggestion is that—like any other life program you may encounter on your journey—you take what you like and leave the rest behind. The key is to listen closely to your own heart and act accordingly.)

As you have discovered by reading my odyssey with constipation, I have been around the block a few times. And from my long, painful years of research, I have discovered a solution that turns me into a major superstar and success story (in my view, anyway) nearly every single morning.

As it turns out, the doctor who prescribed the kefir enemas was an asset to me after all. It was he who casually handed me a tiny pamphlet on managing constipation From those simple guidelines and my own intuition and study, I have come up with a winning combination for bountiful bowel movements, which I humbly share with you.

Here is a brief list of bowel movement components, with fuller explanations to follow:

1. **Eat breakfast first thing in the morning.**
2. **Drink hot liquids (tea, decaf) after breakfast.**
3. **Stay very quiet and calm until bowels move.**
4. **Always respond to an urge from your bowels.**
5. **Drink plenty of water throughout the day.**
6. **Eat foods conducive to bowel movements.**
7. **Avoid foods that cause constipation.**
8. **Do not take laxatives.**
9. **Get enough rest.**
10. **Do exercise daily that moves the bowels.**

(Note: For best results, this routine should accompany a lifestyle of inner freedom, self-expression and love. See Chapters 1 through 19 of this book for guidance and encouragement.)

And now for the details.

1. Breakfast

As many of us know, and as all people with regular bowel movements know, eating stimulates the bowels. And in a healthy body, it really does work. I actually never knew this during my long years of constipation hell. The only thing that got my bowels moving was laxatives or other extreme measures. (See Appendix A: An Odyssey Through Constipation Hell.)

Once we cease and desist from crippling our bodies with laxatives, and follow a few other time-tested practices, our bowels really will be affected by this simple act of eating.

2. Drink hot liquids (tea, decaf, etc.)

Again, this is part of common bowel movement wisdom. As Gore Vidal said, "First coffee, then a bowel movement, then the muse joins me." I drink hot tea and decaf. Regular coffee works wonderfully for this. However, caffeine, which is a very potent drug that I'm surprised is even legal, separates us from our deepest selves. But any hot liquid you choose will work, whether taken after breakfast, or taken upon rising.

3. Quiet time

Here is the heart of the Zen of glorious bowel movements. You may have guessed from the underlining that I consider this to be the most important part of the program. You are right. For me, this is the one critical act that allows my bowels to move every morning. I may, and have, broken some of my own rules, but this one I try never to break.

Why? Because my bowels will not move unless I remain quiet and calm. For instance, even after all these years of daily miracles, I have never, unless I had some sickness like the flu, had a bowel movement after leaving the house. Something happens to my guts when I get out in the world; I tighten up inside and no further bowel action happens.

Sometimes when I am out with friends who have just eaten breakfast, they will jump up and run to the restroom to have their release. I am sick with envy. These people have no idea how wonderful that seems to me; they've been regular all their lives.

That said, I must tell you that having this quiet time—it usually takes from 30 minutes to an hour, sometimes longer, for my bowels to move after breakfast—has been the cornerstone of my spiritual growth. (For more encouragement, see Chapter 9, "Taking Time for Quiet.")

4. Respond to the urge

This important suggestion is symbolic of becoming a fully realized human being—to move with our inner urges. So many of us learned before the age of one to hold back our feces, to hold back our passions, to hold back our deep desires. By the time I reach kindergarten, I was holding back so much I was almost paralyzed. What made me such a "good" child, family members later told me, is that I was so quiet they never knew I was around. Oh, great.

As we learn to listen to and respond to our bodies in the quiet of the morning (or any other time), we can take this habit out into the world. With practice, we can get an urge from our inner selves, trust it, and act on it. We were each brought here to offer special gifts to the world, and I say the world needs us to stop holding back—with our bowel movements and with ourselves. (For further encouragement, see Chapter 5, "Being Authentic," and Chapter 13, "Giving from an Overflowing Cup."

5. Drink lots of water

Again, a perusing of bowel management books will show that keeping the body and bowels well hydrated is key to bowel movement success. It figures that if our insides are all dried up, it will be harder for the body to eliminate. This habit of drinking a lot of water came slowly for me, especially because I took a lot of laxatives for a while and drinking water didn't seem to be necessary for bowel movements then.

But now that my body is using its own powers to move wastes out of itself, it needs water to do the job. I have learned that if I'm trying to drink tap water, which tastes unpleasant (at least where I live in Santa Barbara), I will tend not to drink much water. Therefore, I drink bottled water only and actually enjoy it. It's definitely habit forming. Also, I don't drink water with meals because it dilutes my digestive juices. Rather, I eat a lot of fresh fruits and vegetables, which have the moisture I need during my meal.

For me, giving my body the water it needs to work properly is the first step in giving my whole being what it needs to fully bloom. For instance, I need to be around people who love me just the way I am. If you want to call me needy, go ahead. I have my needs, and I get them met. Otherwise, I have nothing to give back.

6. Eat foods for bowel movement success

What I have found through many years of research is that, for bowel movement ecstasy, my body needs to have a lot of raw vegetables. So I eat a large salad at lunch and dinner. Believe me, I'm not into spending hours on preparing my meals. But I insist on the highest quality food possible. I also eat a lot of fresh, cooked vegetables.

When I stopped eating processed and fast foods, my desire for cooked vegetables developed. Now, I can think of few richer experiences that eating steaming Swiss chard or baked spaghetti squash with a bit of sesame oil. We're talking heaven on Earth here.

One friend of mine believes religiously in eating greens every day—collard greens, mustard greens or turnip greens. They are sold fresh at most markets (at least in Southern California) and frozen in some markets. Again, taking into one's body these rich, nurturing vegetables speaks volumes more of self-love than an entire book of affirmations. As Santa Barbara psychologist David Richo says, you gain self-esteem by acting with self-respect. Another way of saying it is that you don't feel your way into right action. You act your way into right feeling.

(**Important note**: From my reading, I understand that switching to a diet which includes lots of raw vegetables can cause intestinal distress. Please pay attention to yourself and get the help you need from health practitioners. Again, this is my own program only and may not be the answer to your challenges.)

Another food which I absolutely love is plain yogurt. Can you believe that? When I first tried yogurt as a child, I was repulsed. Then, it was the epitome of yucky foods. Now, I can't (excuse me, choose not to) hardly go a day without the stuff. My favorite by yards is Maya plain yogurt, which is hard to find. Other people prefer to eat lowfat or nonfat yogurt and some prefer a yogurt that is less sour that Maya. Having talked about the joy of the taste, let me add that yogurt also has in it certain good bacteria that many people believe we need in our intestines for natural bowel movements. The doctor who prescribed the kefir enemas I mentioned in Appendix A was aiming toward this goal. But I feel that eating yogurt every day is doing the job in a much more pleasant way. Trust me on this one.

7. Avoid foods that cause bowel failure

Coming to understand which foods clog me up has been a very personal thing. Through the years, I have read about foods that are suspected of causing constipated and have experimented to see if that was true for me. This is not a quick process and the tendency is strong to forget the damaging effects of certain otherwise desirable foods and give them one more chance.

The first food I must mention is cheese, which I had been gorging myself with for years. I learned this habit from one family member who ate more cheese during my childhood than anyone I've ever known. This is the same person who found it necessary to take laxatives as a part of her daily life. There is a connection.

These days, I avoid cheese. I consider it a bad food

for me. It binds my system up and no matter how much I adhere to the rest of my bowel movement program, I will be woefully constipated if I eat cheese. It's just not worth it. I won't even give it to my dog. Some pet experts say not to feed cheese to dogs because it causes them constipation. Again, I learn about life from my dog. (See Chapter 17, "Getting a Dog.")

However, I have discovered soy cheese, which tastes to me like the real thing and which my body likes quite well, although some people have difficulty digesting soy products.

Another food that doesn't work for me is milk. I guess I'm allergic to it, which I understand is true for many human adults. Some say adult bodies don't produce the digestive enzymes necessary to break milk down. But sometimes, even this far into my recovery from constipation, I will do what I call "The Milk Experiment," and have a little of the luscious white liquid that reminds me of what motherly love must feel like.

Just minutes after digesting milk, I will get bad gas pains and will start to get a pasty film on my skin. Plus, and this is the worst offense a food can make, I get constipated.

Another food which causes me to clog up is white flour. Many people feel that foods like pasta are the best thing for bowel movement success, but for me they are deleterious. For me, white-flour products turn into a total, bowel-clogging disaster. It turns into some kind of glue that brings my system to a halt and causes me to feel tired and depressed. Again, this is only for me. I offer these words to help you see that your own body will give you the answers. With enough patience and willingness, you can hear the truth, believe it, and act upon it in your own best interest.

8. No laxatives

This is one suggestion that can strike fear in the hearts of those of us who have come to rely on laxatives for any modicum of bowel-movement success. The fear is that we may, without laxatives, never have a bowel movement again. And it has taken me many years of constipation recovery to really adhere to a policy of not taking laxatives.

In the beginning of my constipation recovery, just one day without a bowel movement would seem like the beginning of a long period of constipation and I would go ahead and take a laxative. But now I know—and I sort of knew then—that taking laxatives reduces my chances of having a normal bowel movement any time in the near future. It takes my body days and weeks to get back its own strength and internal muscle tone after a bout with laxatives.

But what about the laxative companies who are only trying to make an honest living? Here, again, is where we can listen to our own bodies and let them be our directors. (See Chapter 6, "Keeping Outside Images in Their Place") for more encouragement.) I, of all people, know how hard it is to live through a constipated day without surrendering to chemicals. My standard rule in the beginning of my bowel recovery, before my body was accustomed to eliminating every morning, was to endure at least three days of constipation before taking laxatives.

I'm not into self-abuse, by any means, and would not want to wait a week or more before having a bowel movement. But I needed to give my body a chance to right itself. And the three-days rule typically did the trick; I would usually have a major release before the deadline was upon me.

These days, it's more subtle. One day I might not have as full a bowel movement as I would like, and then the next day's release will more than make up for it. Most of all, I want to honor my body and not set it back in its recovery by forcing it to perform with chemicals.

9. Get enough rest

After my long term of study, I've found that my body and bowels need rest before they will function properly. This is again the Zen of the program, letting the body function as it truly wants and needs to. My body has requirements for smooth operation, like a car need regular oil changes. Rest is one of those necessities. Like the other suggestions in this chapter, this one is important to me and may not have any bearing on your own situation. It's one more thing for you to think about, experiment with, and possibly adopt as a part of your life.

According to some articles I've read lately, we are a nation of sleep-deprived people. There's so much stimulation—things to do, people to see, goals to accomplish, bosses to please. For some of us, such busy, non-stop lives are not conducive to the fantastic bowel movements we need to be healthy. (For encouragement, see Chapter 3, "Living a Simple, Sacred Life.")

10. Exercise

Here is another part of my program that has taken me many years to adopt. Without some pretty amazing motivation, exercise for me can be hell. Especially when I haven't exercised for a few weeks or months (or years!), the thought of exercise turns my stomach (but unfortunately doesn't stimulate my bowels!)

But daily exercise is necessary for naturally occurring bowel movements, as I have found in my own experience and read in countless books. The good thing is, once I have a routine going, it feels fantastic to exercise.

But I am easy on myself, too. Since I started living a

life of following my my inner wisdom, I notice that on some days I have low energy and feel soft and reflective. On those days, I don't force myself to do strenuous exercise. I still move my body, but more slowly and without pressure. A walk usually sounds good at these times. On other days, I feel like conquering the world and I go for it, practically running up the mountain trails behind my home.

To build the muscle tone necessary for stupendous bowel movements, exercises that move the abdominal area are best. Among these are walking, hiking, jogging, swimming and working out on the step machine. Yoga is another fabulous way to move all parts of the body and there are ancient yogic exercises which are expressly designed to bring about a mind-blowing bowel movement.

When I first realized I would need to exercise daily (for bowel management and to combat depression), I joined the local YMCA and worked out on the step machine every day. Now I go hiking in the mountains almost every day.

This form of exercise includes two of my passions: being with my wonderful dog, Molly, and being with my true mother, the Earth. In order to want to exercise, we must find something we love. If we were born to need exercise, we were also born with a deep passion for some kind of movement.

Conclusion

This is a program that works for me. Your program will be different. And I certainly don't make any claim to perfection in my own practice. But I know that my adherence to the above principles is directly proportional to my luck in the morning, and my comfort level the rest of the day. As I mentioned above, and which I can't express enough, this physical program must go hand-in-hand with a spiritual and emotional program of being our true, authentic selves.

For if we are holding back who we really are as humans, we can't expect our bodies to do otherwise.

To order more copies of
"The Zen of Bowel Movements,"
send $19.95 plus $3 shipping and handling
for each copy to:

Rock Rose Publishing
P.O. Box 192
Santa Barbara, CA 93102
Phone: (805) 969-2158